THE FUTURE PATIENT

Liz Kendall

ippr

30-32 Southampton St
London WC2E 7RA
Tel: 020 7470 6100
Fax: 020 7470 6111
postmaster@ippr.org.uk
www.ippr.org
Registered charity 800065

The Institute for Public Policy Research is an independent charity whose purpose is to contribute to public understanding of social, economic and political questions through research, discussion and publication. It was established in 1988 by leading figures in the academic, business and trade-union communities to provide an alternative to the free market think tanks.

IPPR's research agenda reflects the challenges facing Britain and Europe. Current programmes cover the areas of economic and health policy, governmental reform, human rights, social policy, the environment and media issues.

Besides its programme of research and publication, IPPR also provides a forum for political and trade union leaders, academic experts and those from business, finance, government and the media, to meet and discuss issues of common concern.

Production & design by **EMPHASIS**
ISBN 1 86030 175 4

Contents

Acknowledgements

I would like to thank the members of the Future Patient Advisory Group for all their help and advice during the course of the project. They include: Angela Coulter, Picker Institute, Europe; Anne Damerell, Pain Concern; Dr Simon Fradd, British Medical Association; Bob Gann, NHS Direct Online; Pippa Gough, King's Fund; Angela Hayes, International Association of Patients' Organisations; Susan Lewis, Gauches Association; Clara McKay, Consumers' Association; Sir Alexander Macara, National Heart Forum and University of York; Gopa Mitra, Proprietary Association of Great Britain; Barrie Taylor, CHC's Development Association; Matthew Taylor, IPPR and Kate Tillett, Merck Sharp and Dohme.

I would also like to thank all those who participated in a recent seminar to discuss an earlier draft of this report for their comments and suggestions. I am particularly grateful to Helena Scott and Lisa Harker from IPPR for their valuable help in producing this report.

This project has been made possible due to the generous support of Merck Sharp & Dohme

About the author

Liz Kendall is the Senior Research Fellow in Health Policy at IPPR. She was previously the Fellow of the Public Health Programme at the King's Fund (1998-2000) and Special Adviser to Harriet Harman, MP (1996-1998). Liz's publications include: *Citizens' Juries* (IPPR, 1994), *Local Inequalities Targets* (King's Fund, 1999), *Improving London's Health: The role of the Greater London Authority* (King's Fund, 2000) and *The Report of the Policy Forum on the Future of Health and Health Care* (IPPR, 2000).

1. Introduction

The past decade has seen many policies which have sought to ensure the NHS becomes a more patient-centred service, from the last Conservative Government's Patient Charter to the current Government's NHS Plan which makes much of the need to modernise services 'around the needs of patients'. Yet despite these efforts, the rhetoric of a patient-centred health service often fails to materialise in reality. Whilst official patient surveys consistently show high levels of satisfaction with the NHS, delve beneath the surface and a very different picture emerges. Many patients do talk about receiving an excellent standard of care from the NHS. When things go well, patients are seen quickly, channels of communication are clear and the patient finds their way through the system with ease and confidence. The key factor determining whether patients feel they have had a good experience is the way they have been treated by health professionals. Patients want to be given enough time and information, to be listened to and have all their questions answered and, crucially, to be treated as individual.

However, more often than not the typical patient experience within the NHS is not perceived as good. Patients frequently talk about their experiences as frustrating, time consuming and even frightening. It is often the detail of the experience that contributes to a poor encounter: being put on a mixed ward, having dirty sheets or getting different or conflicting views from different health professionals. By far the biggest problem patients face is waiting. Patients feel they have to wait too long at every stage of their treatment. Time spent with health professionals is a precious commodity and one that is in increasingly short supply. Patients often fell powerless in what is seen as an increasingly bureaucratic and cumbersome system. Experiences within the NHS are often described as confrontations, with patients feeling they have to struggle with the service to get what they want out of it, from getting past the 'difficult' receptionist in their local GP's surgery to understanding the complicated language doctors use to explain conditions and treatments. Patients feel they constantly have to pester people to get the information or help they need. Individual doctors and nurses working within the NHS are frequently described in glowing terms, however patients often characterise their relationship with the NHS as a whole as a battle between 'them and us'.

Whilst personal experiences of the health service are by no means entirely negative, patients generally see the NHS as a service which is under pressure, under resourced and under staffed. There is a keen sense that the NHS is being stretched to its limits with staff being expected to work long hours for low wages. Media coverage of criminal or negligent doctors means patients are beginning to question the almost blind faith they once had in health professionals. Patients' outlook about the future of the NHS is generally pessimistic. Whilst the vast majority want the NHS to continue, they feel it is on a 'slippery slope' and that things will inevitably become worse in future.

The NHS is already going through major changes which seek to ensure it becomes more genuinely 'patient-centred'. New services like NHS Direct and walk in centres aim to provide patients with more flexible access to advice and treatment. Collaborative programmes on cancer and primary care are seeking to redesign services 'around the needs of patients' as are measures to ensure closer working between health and social care. The NHS Plan also sets out a range of proposals to ensure patients' views are more effectively heard throughout the NHS, including a new Patient Advocacy and Liaison Service and Patients Forums in every hospital and primary care trust to provide direct patient input into how local services are run.

However, more profound challenges to the ways in which health services are organised and experienced are already on the horizon. Developments in information technology are opening up new ways of delivering and accessing services. The human genome project is increasing our understanding of the role genetics plays in disease, creating new opportunities for diagnosis and treatment. These and other technological advances are influencing, and influenced by, wider changes in society where patients are increasingly informed and less deferential and where knowledge is no longer the sole preserve of health professionals.

A number of analyses of likely future trends in health and healthcare have been produced in recent years.[1] Most of these focus on which trends may be technologically possible and on the attitudes of and implications for professionals and policy makers – not on what current or future patients' views might be. Yet developing an understanding of patients' attitudes towards likely future trends is crucial, not only because they could affect whether and how future developments are implemented but also because of broader democratic and accountability issues.

This report is an attempt to address the current gap in knowledge. It identifies the key trends that are likely to influence health and healthcare over the next five to fifteen years. It outlines what patients want from their health services including their attitudes towards key future developments, drawing in particular on the results of recent qualitative research conducted by IPPR (see Appendix for details). The paper assesses the implications of these views for Government, professionals, industry and patients themselves, and outlines policy proposals based on the emerging analysis.

2. Future trends in health and healthcare

The first section of this paper outlines the key future trends in health and healthcare over the next five to fifteen years. There are clearly a wide range of issues that could be considered here and the aim of this paper is to identify the most important and relevant trends. These are grouped under the following headings:

- Wider changes in society: including the ageing population, evolving family structures and gender relations, the growth in consumerism, and global and environmental factors.
- New health and healthcare technologies: including medical advances like drugs and treatments emerging from the human genome project, and advances in how healthcare and information is delivered, like robotics, the internet and telemedicine.
- The health policy agenda: including quicker, more flexible access to treatment, an increased emphasis on primary care, the further integration of health and social care, and the changing roles of health professionals and patients.

Wider changes in society

There are many layers of influence on an individual's health. Firstly, fixed factors which individuals are endowed with such as age, gender and genetics. Secondly, individual lifestyle factors – the personal behaviour and way of life individuals adopt which can damage or promote health. Thirdly, social and community influences such as how people interact with friends, relatives and their immediate community which can help sustain the health of community members in otherwise unfavourable conditions. Fourthly, the living and working conditions encountered as part of daily life such as access to food supplies and essential services. Finally, the broader socio-economic, cultural and environmental conditions which can have a bearing on every other layer of influence. These include the standard of living of particular groups (which can influence individual eating, drinking, smoking and exercise habits) and eliefs, such as views about the place of women in society or attitudes towards ethnic minority groups (Dahlgren and Whitehead, 1991). The following analysis is based on this socio-economic model of health.

Demographic issues

Perhaps one of the most important factors influencing the future health of the nation is the UK's ageing population.[2] By 2015, life expectancy is predicted to increase to 77 years for men and 83 years for women.[3] By 2036 it is estimated that there will be seven million people over seventy years old, up from 4.3 million at present. One of the major consequences of the UK's ageing population is that the total long term care bill is expected to rise from around £12 billion at present to £34.5 billion by 2030 (Dargie, 1999).

Whilst further research on the disease profile associated with an ageing population is required, some broad trends are already clear. The UK, like other industrialised countries, is likely to experience a relative decline in the burden of communicable, maternal, peri-natal and nutritional conditions and a shift to chronic, non-communicable diseases including diabetes, hypertension and cardiovascular disease. As people live longer, a higher prevalence of cancer is expected. By 2018, lung cancer and breast cancer will pose the largest disease burden for women, and prostate, colon and lung cancer will pose the largest burden for men (East Anglian Cancer Intelligence Unit, 1997). A 'life-course' approach to the likely future disease burden has identified two key trends.[4] Firstly, an increase in smoking related diseases, particularly amongst women, including lung cancer, emphysema and chronic bronchitis. Secondly, an increase in the prevalence of asthma because of the rising asthma and allergy rates currently seen amongst children and adolescents (Dargie, 1999). The effects of smoking on the future health of the population are unclear. Until recently it was expected that male lung cancer would decline because of the reduction in the proportion of men smoking but that female lung cancer would increase because of the increasing number of women, particularly young women, who currently smoke. However recent figures have shown a worrying increase in smoking rates amongst both men and women.

Several other likely trends in the future disease burden have been identified. The World Health Organisation has suggested that social and psychological ill health may increase in future (WHO, 1998). This could be a conequence of the increase in stress caused by modern lifestyles in industrialised countries (see below) and a decrease in the stigma of reporting mental ill health. Recent reports from both the Chief Medical Officer (Calman, 1998) and the British Council (British Council, 1998) have predicted an increase in obesity, due to the poor diet and reduced exercise, which again may be caused by 21st century lifestyles in western countries.

Evolving family structures and gender relations

Families have an important influence on health, both in terms of the care they have traditionally provided for children and disabled, elderly or sick relatives and the wider health benefits that are associated with social networks (see below). It is predicted that more people will be living alone over the coming decades. Whereas the biggest group of people living alone is currently women aged over 60 years old, the largest increase in recent years has been men aged under 65 years, reflecting the decline in marriage and rise in separation and divorce. It is predicted that men under 65 years will overtake older women as the largest group of single person households within the next ten years. Although the number of single parent families has grown, most dependent children still live in families with two parents, in part due to the increase in the number of step-families.

Fertility rates are currently rising for older women and falling for younger women as childbirth is delayed. Delaying childbirth could affect healthcare provision in future, for example by increasing demand for services like IVF. Predictions about future fertility rates differ. Some commentators suggest that overall fertility rates will rise from 1.72 children per woman in 1998 to 1.8 in 2015. Others expect a fall in overall fertility rates: those women who decide to have children will give birth to an average of two children, but the 25 per cent of women who are expected to remain childless (through choice or otherwise) could bring the overall average down to 1.5 children per woman (Dargie, 1999).

Evolving gender roles at home and at work could have an impact on the health of the population. Women are increasingly gaining professional and technical qualifications and entering high paid careers. The higher financial rewards that employment brings could have a beneficial impact on women's health. However, the increase in the number of mothers in the workplace could also expose women to greater levels of stress as they struggle to balance work and family responsibilities. More women are affected by relationship breakdown or are choosing to live alone and bring up their children independently. Lone parents are particularly prone to ill health, even after controlling for household income, employment status and occupation, which may in part be a result of the stigma traditionally associated with being a lone parent (Coote and Kendall, 2000). Men's health may also be affected by changing gender roles. One reason for the increase in suicide rates amongst young men could be the erosion of traditional notions of masculinity. The restructuring of the labour market has led to fewer 'masculine' jobs and unemployment may be more of a blow to self-esteem for men than for women, at least as long as the traditional male role as family breadwinner persists (Pahl 1999).

It has been argued that in understanding the causes of ill health we need to consider how social and economic change affects gender and how changing gender roles affect health (Coote and Kendall, 2000). As paid employment becomes more significant to the identity of women, will unemployment carry a greater health risk for them? If men play a greater role in parenting, deriving from it an enhanced sense of purpose and identity, could that mean they will find it easier to cope with spells of unemployment? As lone parenthood becomes more commonplace and less stigmatised, is it less likely to be correlated with ill health in women?

Social networks

Evidence is emerging about the influence of social networks on health. A social network is the set of personal contacts through which people maintain their social identity and receive emotional support, material aid, information on services and new social contacts. This network may include relatives, friends, neighbours and fellow employees. The quality of relationships in this 'micro-social world' is increasingly seen as having a vital role to play in achieving and maintaining better health (Putnam, 2001). However, the impact of social networks on health and healthcare is highly complex and often contradictory. Some research has found that close-knit social networks are associated with longer delays in contacting health services, whilst other studies show they lead to more ready use. A study in the 1970s found that people who underused antenatal services were more likely than those who used the service to be living with members of their family. More recent research has highlighted the importance of the telephone for maintaining long distance family ties and providing social support, suggesting that geographical proximity may not be as important as it was in the past (Rogers, Hassell and Nicolaas, 1999). The types of social networks people experience are clearly changing. Family ties have traditionally been seen as offering greater material assistance and long-term commitment, with people being more reluctant to rely on friends than family members for continuing support and care. However, friends and friend-like relations are arguably becoming more salient in contemporary society (Pahl, 1999). This is partly due to geographical and social mobility, which makes it more difficult for traditional family supports to be maintained.

Whilst the links between socio-economic factors and health are well established (see below), it is not yet clearly understood how and why certain personal communities are more effective than others. More people may be getting divorced, living alone, and moving around country. Will this lead to a decrease in attachment and subsequent negative impact on health or might these trends in fact lead to an increase in attachment because of a new focus on friendship? Are 'friend' rich communities healthier than 'friend poor' communities? If so, what are the processes and mechanisms involved? Is society becoming more or less friendly and what are the likely future trends?

Modern lifestyles and the growth in consumerism

We live in an increasingly wealthy and consumerist society. Services that were previously open during the traditional nine to five working week are now available around the clock. People are becoming more informed and less deferential. There has been an explosion of information available over the internet, increasing numbers of people are entering further or higher education and there are more media outlets than ever before with news now accessible twenty four hours a day. People's expectations for their own health and quality of life are rising, as are their expectations about health services and the people who deliver them. The paternalism long associated with the health service is also being eroded, in part due to recent high profile cases about 'dangerous doctors' like Harold Shipman and Rodney Ledward.

An increasingly wealthy and consumerist society may have important consequences for the future health of the population. As people become increasingly educated, they may be more aware of the benefits of healthy living. On the other hand, an increase in disposable income could lead to more opportunities for drinking, overeating and drug taking. There has been a growth in the number of 'work rich: time poor' and 'work poor: time rich' households. People who have jobs are working increasingly longer hours and travelling longer distances to work. The amount of quality time people have to spend with their families is declining. Rates of divorce are increasing and the growth in step-families means already scarce family time may have to be more widely shared (Pahl, 199). Even though job security may not be objectively less than in the past, the end of a job for life appears to have increased feelings of insecurity. Sociologists like Beck and Giddens argue that we are living in a 'risk society' where people are more anxious about food, the environment, global warming, the dangers of travel and a whole host of other real or imagined dangers and disasters (Beck, 1992). These developments may have an important bearing on the psychological health and well-being of the population.

The prevailing view is that the wealthier society becomes the more demanding patients will be, but it is important to question whether there may in fact be limits to consumerist tendencies within the NHS. Some research suggests people see healthcare, particularly medicines, as fundamentally different from other sorts of 'consumer' goods. One consequence of this view is that support for the role of health professionals as gatekeepers to care appears to remain strong (IPPR, 1998). Patients may not see themselves simply as individuals with a right to 'consume' as much healthcare as they want. They are often acutely aware of the needs of others in the NHS and frequently state that they try not to bother their GP with minor complaints and instead try to deal with the problem at home or by seeking help from pharmacists (Hassell *et al*, 1997). Patients often express concern about taking up too much of hospital doctors' time when other patients need to be seen and when the NHS is facing increasing pressure to ration care. Patients are also aware of the condition others are in, for example if older patients are not eating their food in hospital. Patients seem less willing to tolerate incidents of poor care of others even when they are reluctant to complain about their own treatment (Boudioni and McPherson, 2000).

It is important not to over-stress this point. The above evidence suggests that patients may not act in an entirely consumerist way because of the poor state of the NHS at present. If the system as a whole improves, more egalitarian and altruistic attitudes towards the use of services could change as patients perceive there is less of a need to constrain their demands. Furthermore, if Government policy stresses only individual patients' 'rights' to healthcare and fails to develop an understanding of which reciprocal responsibilities might be expected to have in return, the all demanding, 'consumerist' model of healthcare could become a reality further down the line. (This point is discussed in greater detail in the concluding section of this report.)

Poverty and inequality

The UK as a whole may be becoming richer, but not everyone shares fairly in the country's rising prosperity. Poverty blights the lives of too many people living in the country, yet this fact is frequently overlooked by those gazing into the 'crystal ball' of future healthcare trends:

> Perhaps the greatest danger of all [ie to the future health of the population] is that generated by poverty... The futurologists with an over great faith in the combination of economic growth and the technological fix are not always ready to accept that socially damaging levels of inequality are likely to persist (Pahl 1999).

There is clear evidence that people who live in disadvantaged circumstances have more illnesses, more disability and shorter lives than those who are more affluent. People in social classes IV and V live on average five years less than those in social classes I and II. If death rates for men aged under 65 years in the most disadvantaged groups were the same as those in the most advantaged groups, there would be 17,000 fewer deaths each year (Independent Inquiry into Inequalities in Health, 1998). Wilkinson argues that it is not absolute but relative poverty that has a fundamental impact on levels of social and physical health and well-being, and that the evidence strongly suggests the health benefits of more cohesive and egalitarian societies (Wilkinson, 1996). It is not just a matter of having the money to purchase life's essentials that is important. People's feelings of self-esteem and self-worth also bear heavily on their health. Those in more egalitarian societies and in less hierarchically structured institutions are likely to have more sense of personal control over what they do and how they present themselves to others, and this in turn may help to reduce anxiety. Britain is a highly unequal country. Whether this situation will change in future is hotly contested. For example, income inequality has grown substantially since 1979 and latest figures suggest it continues to do so (Economic Trends, 2001). However, it has been argued that there is a substantial time lag in the official statistics and that the impact of measures being implemented by the current Government, such as the Working Families Tax Credit and increases in Child Benefit and children's rates in Income Support will not become apparent in the official statistics until 2002 (Hills 2001).

Global and environmental trends

It has already been suggested that the future disease burden in industrialised countries is likely to focus on chronic, non-communicable diseases. However, some commentators have warned of the possible emergence or re-emergence of infectious diseases as a major challenge to health. In future, antibiotic-resistant infections, HIV and food borne diseases could all come to the fore because of the increasingly global context within which health is experienced and delivered (Dargie 1999).

The greater mobility of people, animals, plants, goods and services across national boundaries could all lead to a rise in the number of diseases entering the UK. An increasingly global health market could lead to threats from goods that are detrimental to ill health being more freely traded such as tobacco, alcohol, junk food, prostitution and illicit drugs. Foodborne diseases may be more easily transmissible (both into and out of the country) because of the food industry's worldwide system of manufacture, storage and distribution. BSE is the most prominent example of a trans-border health risk from food in recent years (Lee, 1999). Diseases like malaria could become more common because of increased travel to tropical countries. Climate change could also have an impact. Palmer has argued: 'Whilst there may be positive health outcomes resulting from the increase in global temperatures, for example decreased mortality from cold related respiratory disease, the net public health impact of climate change will probably be negative'. The number of people suffering from skin cancer or eye lesions (cataracts) could increase through exposure to ultra violet radiation from a depleted ozone layer. An increase in urban air pollution could result in a rising incidence of cardio-respiratory deaths. However, the importance of outdoor pollution should not be over-stated as its impact on health is likely to be small in comparison with the affect of the indoor environment such as poor housing or smoking (Palmer 1999).

Globalisation will not only affect the sorts of diseases that might be experienced in future: it could also affect the ways in which people access health information, care and services. The internet, telemedicine, and greater opportunities for travel may expose UK patients to different health systems and to products or services which may be unavailable in this country. This could clearly heighten patients' expectations and demands, presenting a major challenge to national governments (as was seen with the recent case of the drug Viagra). The internet could promote both healthy and unhealthy lifestyles and lead to products of dubious and even potentially harmful effect being sold worldwide. It could also increase the recognition of alternative medicines, like Chinese medicine and homeopathy, challenging the dominance and spread of Western biomedicine worldwide (Lee, 1999).

Technological drivers of change

Some important caveats must be made before analysing the likely future technological drivers of change. Firstly, no-one can predict with certainty all the new health technologies the next five to fifteen years will bring. It has been suggested that: 'in the area of scientific and technological discoveries...future projections are often over optimistic about what will be discovered by when and make unrealistic assumptions about the implementation of discoveries in everyday use' (Robert 1999). This is because too often the focus is on what is technically possible, not what is socially or ethically acceptable: human values and needs cannot and must not be ignored when looking at what might happen in future. Indeed, some commentators suggest that there seems to be a growing public fear of technology per se, often because of an accompanying perceived neglect of personal care. Qualitative research supports this analysis. Patients and the wider public expect 'technology' to be a key feature of the healthcare world of the future. There is a sense of inevitably about this development and a grudging acceptance that 'technology' is the way forward. However, patients voice deep concerns about the implications that certain technologies could bring (Edwards, 2001).

Secondly, any assessment of likely future trends in healthcare must acknowledge the potential for the unexpected. As Marinker argues, what tends to be missing from most future clinical scenarios is the unpredictable – the fundamental challenges to present assumptions about science in general and healthcare in particular: 'What has gone before inevitably influences where to look next and what to recognise, but it cannot accommodate surprise' (Marinker 1998).

Bearing these points in mind, future technological drivers are grouped under two broad headings in the following section. The first covers developments in bioengineering, transplantation, new lifestyle drugs and genetics – what might loosely be called 'medical advances'. The second focuses more on advances in *how* health care and information might be delivered, such as image guided surgery, robotics and new information and communication technologies like the internet and telemedicine.

Medical advances

Bioengineering

As people live longer, the demand for existing implants like hip replacements is likely to grow. Demand for other implants such as knee, shoulder and finger joint replacements, heart valves and pacemakers is also set to increase. Many biomaterials (non-biological materials destined for biological venues) that are currently used have a limited patient-lifetime which means repeat operations may be necessary. Bioengineering could help ensure implants last longer in future. Bioengineering applies engineering principles to human biology in areas like cell biology and plastic manufacture. At its simplest, the idea is to make organs rather than to move them. Examples include tissue engineering: living cells combined with biologically friendly synthetic polymers which ultimately dissolve, leaving behind new versions of functioning biological tissue bearing no trace of non-biological material. It has been predicted that electronic implants to stimulate muscles in disabled people could be available by 2002, artificial hearts by 2010, and artificial senses (using sensors which stimulate nerves), kidneys and lungs by 2015 (Robert, 1999).

Transplantation

The major challenges facing transplantation are limited organ availability and the fact that the effectiveness of transplants continues to be limited by rejection. Future developments are likely to include immunosuppressive drugs that are more effective and specific, and less toxic. This could lead to organs and tissues like the pancreas and endocrine organs being successfully transplanted. Skin cloning and the growth of retinol tissue may also be successfully developed. Organ and tissue replacements of the future could more often combine living tissue with some artificial components. The need for organ donors will continue to increase as more and new diseases become eligible for treatment by transplant. It is unlikely there will ever be enough human organ donors to meet demand and xenografts – organs from other species – offer a potential solution. Several biotech companies are already investing in developing genetically modified animals (Robert, 1999). However, major concerns about the possibility of trans-species diseases will have be overcome before the use of this technology is accepted, particularly in the wake of diseases like BSE and vCJD.

Lifestyle drugs

Future medical advances could provide cures for many existing diseases. One consequence could be an increase in the number of so-called 'lifestyle' drugs that are available. Current lifestyle drugs include Viagra for impotence and Propecia for baldness. These drugs could present major challenges for the NHS.[5] It has been argued that lifestyle drugs treat conditions, or elements of conditions, with characteristics which may not necessarily include ill-health. Unlike many types of ill health, problems such as obesity, impotence and baldness derive some (if not all) of their significance from the person's inability to act satisfactorily in social situations. The conditions which lifestyle drugs treat are certainly unfortunate, unpleasant, unwanted, irritating or even worse. But are they 'ill-health'? If not, should they be the concern of the NHS?

Lifestyle drugs are only one example of a whole range of services linked by the same sense of uncertainty as to their place in a national, publicly funded health service. For example, are people who cannot have children suffering from ill health? If not, should IVF treatment be available on the NHS? The NHS is already struggling to deal with these issues and an increase in lifestyle drugs could magnify the problem. Establishing effective mechanisms to define which conditions or ailments are considered to constitute 'ill health' could become a major challenge in future (Peckham, 1998).

Genetics

One of the most important developments likely to affect future patients is the new genetics.[6] Clinicians and commentators disagree about the likely pace and nature of change genetics will bring. Enthusiasts believe medicine as it is currently practised will change completely within the next five to fifteen years. Advances in knowledge about the human genome will affect not only the treatment and management of rare single gene disorders such as cystic fibrosis or sickle cell disease but also more common disorders including diabetes, cancer, cardiovascular disease, arthritis and asthma. Others suggest that assessing the precise contribution of genes to particular diseases is likely remain highly problematic and that knowledge about genetics will not necessarily translate into opportunities for more effective prevention or treatment. These more cautious voices maintain that the future practice of medicine will change very little from now and that even if a paradigm shift is to take place, the 'genetic revolution' is still a long way off.

In spite of such conflicting views, the underlying potential of knowledge emerging from the human genome project is clear: 'Few would question that recent developments in genetics will prove to be the most significant scientific advances of the current era and it is inevitable that this will eventually feed through to affect many, if not all, of clinical medicine' (Bell, 1998). Since the 18th century, diseases have been classified according to their symptoms (the disease *phenotype*) and recognised by their common characteristics, derived from populations of patients, from averages and composites of individual examples. Diagnoses based on this approach, whilst clearly useful in the past, inevitably lack precision. The new genetics could lead to a very different, more precise and profound level of diagnosis and therefore treatment. Increasing knowledge about the *genotype* (the genetic make up of a cell or individual) is likely to improve understanding about the biochemical or physiological causes of disease. Since many treatments have tended to concentrate on relieving the symptoms rather than addressing the causes of disease, a better understanding of disease mechanisms could enable a more rational approach to the development of treatments and therapies.

Drugs may increasingly be designed to fit the specific molecular processes involved in causing disease and be targeted at those most likely to benefit. Genetic testing or screening could offer the potential to identify at-risk individuals with opportunities for preventative measures such as education about lifestyle changes and monitoring for earlier diagnosis and treatment. It is not only more personalised and effective drugs that could be seen in the coming years, but also new types of treatment such as gene therapy: the replacement or repair of defective genes in living cells. Some commentators predict that drugs and treatments emerging from the human genome project will be the key driver of increased costs of healthcare in future: 'In the years to come, technological developments [will] be the most important of the pressures on health service costs, of which genetic technologies [are] likely to provide one of the most challenging examples' (Zimmern and Cook, 2000). However, others refute this position. For example, Bell has suggested: 'The current system is ineffective because of lack of precision, and if that precision can be gleaned effectively...then the economic benefits are likely to be real'. For example, the cost of drug development is likely to fall because drug development programmes will be more likely to achieve success because of appropriate patient selection and stratification (Bell, 1998).

It must be acknowledged that many of the above developments have so far proved more elusive than early enthusiasts predicted, particularly gene therapy. However, if gene therapy is still some way off, the advent of genetic testing is already on the horizon. Genetic tests for single gene disorders such as cystic fibrosis and for susceptibility genes for more common disorders such as cancer and heart disease are likely to become available in the UK over the coming decades. The issue of genetic testing and the consequences for insurance cover has attracted considerable attention to date.[7] To summarise the debate, there is grave concern that individuals who are required to disclose the results of genetic tests to insurance companies will run the risk of being refused cover or asked to pay a disproportionately high premium. Eventually, certain sections of the population could become uninsurable. Furthermore, if insurance companies can insist on disclosure of the results of genetic tests, it could deter people at risk of a disorder from taking the test and, where possible, receiving early treatment. In turn, insurers are concerned about the risk of adverse selection, whereby individuals who believe that they might be at greater risk of suffering from conditions with a genetic element may be more likely to insure themselves for larger amounts if they do not have to share genetic information. Insurance companies can ask for the results of just one genetic test at present – that of Huntington's disease – although the Human Genetics Committee has recently proposed a three year moratorium on genetic testing which the Government has said it will implement.

Advances in healthcare delivery

Diagnostic and monitoring equipment

Advances in healthcare equipment could have a major impact on where care is delivered in future. Desktop analysers could enable chemical pathology and biochemistry tasks to be performed in the local GPs surgery with the results immediately available to doctors and patients, thereby helping to reduce waiting times. The reduced size and portability of diagnostic and treatment equipment means they could be more easily used in local primary care centres or even in patients' homes. Indeed it has been suggested that the home could become the key site of healthcare delivery over the next five to fifteen years (Robert, 1999). The availability of genetic tests and remote diagnostic equipment, such as heart monitors and blood glucose measurement devices, are all likely to contribute to this trend, as are future trends in healthcare policy (see below).

Minimal access and image guided surgery

Other developments are also likely to reduce the reliance on hospitals in future. Developments like endoscopy have already helped to reduce the length of inpatient stays in hospital and to shift the focus of services away from traditional acute hospitals. The Office of Science and Technology's (OST) Foresight Programme has forecast that by 2010 to 2014, 50 per cent of surgery will be conducted through minimal access techniques.

Developments which build on Magnetic Resonance Imaging (MRI) may lead to new forms of image guided surgery in the coming years. This technique aims not just to find out what is wrong with the body but to instruct, guide and even control the surgeon during the operation. Image guided surgery could help surgeons see with better resolution, orientation and context setting: essentially providing vision inside solid objects. Whilst it is unlikely that open surgery will be a thing of the past in twenty years time, it has been predicted that far fewer operations will require long hospital stays and the distinction between surgery, medicine and radiology, as well as between primary and secondary care, will be increasingly blurred (Robert, 1999).

Robotics

The OST's Foresight Programme has also predicted that by 2010 to 2014, as many as ten per cent of operations could be carried out by robotic technicians. The potential benefits of using robotic devices in surgery over humans include greater three dimensional spatial accuracy, especially when linked to scanning technology, the potential for enhanced reliability and the capacity to produce more repeatable outcomes, and a degree of precision far greater than that achievable by human beings. Techniques that could be available over the next ten years include a completely controlled endoscope which can follow its nose to a predefined site thereby avoiding damage to normal tissue. In the USA a robot, aptly named RoboDoc, is already being used to perform total hip replacements. A development related to robotics is telepresence surgery. This enables surgeons to operate at a distance from patients using robots guided by remote control. This technique could also help lead to greater healthcare being available at the primary care level, however it is very much in the experimental stage and unlikely to be more widely available within the next decade (Robert, 1999).

Information and communication technologies

Information and communication technologies could revolutionise healthcare over the next five to fifteen years. The internet could vastly increase opportunities for both patients and doctors to access health information. Email could be used not only to issue repeat prescriptions but also for on-line consultations. Touch screen public information kiosks, digital television and the new generation of mobile phones could help improve access to both services and information. Electronic Health Records (due to be available across the NHS by 2004) will put patients' medical history onto a single 'smart card'. This will enable patients to electronically access their health records and help to ensure greater continuity of care as points of access to the health service expand.

Most assessments of future trends in healthcare predict the increased use of telemedicine as a major factor influencing the organisation, delivery and experience of services. Telemedicine has been defined as the use of telecommunications to provide medical services to distant locations (Mitchell, 2000). It is estimated that there are currently around 120 telemedicine projects in the UK.[8] Examples of telemedicine in this and other countries include video-linking psychiatrists in community mental health centres with general practices in remote areas (May *et al*, 2000), radiologists in local hospitals using video link up to discuss results of radiographs with more qualified specialists in tertiary hospitals (Mitchell 2000), and improving and expanding home care for dialysis patients by using video based support (Stroetmann *et al*, 2000).

Telemedicine could have a major impact on where care is delivered in future, allowing specialist care to be more readily available at the local level, thereby cutting waiting times for treatment and reducing the need to travel particularly in rural areas. It could open up new training opportunities for health professionals and help to improve standards of care. Telemedicine could also be a major driver in enabling and empowering patients to take greater responsibility for their own healthcare. It has been suggested, for example, that telemedicine could ultimately enable patients with diabetes (a disease which is likely to grow in prevalence as the population ages) to take control over the management of their disease, through more effectively self-monitoring their blood glucose levels, examining their feet and so on (Dennis and Owens, 2000).

Modelling the potential impact of future technologies on healthcare systems is notoriously problematic. However, a recent study suggests that telemedicine could lead to major changes in the organisation of health services. It predicts that the number of GP visits could be reduced by 10 to 25 per cent and the number of acute inpatient beds could decline by between 3 to 13 per cent. Conversely, the number of patients monitored at home could increase by between 2,500 and 10,000, community in-patient beds could rise by 10 to 20 per cent and the number of day surgery beds could increase by anywhere between 10 and 50 per cent (Rawlinson, Kelly and Whittlesone, 2000).

It is important to recognise that telemedicine raises issues which cannot be addressed by national governments and professional bodies alone. For example, international standards for the provision of healthcare through telemedicine may need to be developed. But how can commonality and the quality of professional practice be assured across different countries? Which legislative body has precedence and whose standards apply? Where does clinical responsibility lie: with the practitioner in the remote consulting site or the doctor in the specialist tertiary centre? What implications might this have for the regulation of different professionals, and indeed an effective system of complaints?

Health policy agenda

The final driver of change that needs to be considered is the likely future health policy agenda. Clearly, health policies can and do change with different governments. However, there are a number of trends which are likely to continue or increase in future, whichever political party is in power.

Quicker, more flexible access to treatment

Perhaps the most important of these is the drive to cut waiting time for treatment. The current Government, like its predecessor, has put cutting waiting at the top of its agenda for reforming the NHS.[9] By 2004, patients should be able to see a GP within 48 hours. By the end of 2005, maximum waiting times for outpatient appointments will be three months and for inpatient appointments, six months. The private sector is expected to play an increasing role in delivering these commitments. The Concordat that the Government signed with the independent healthcare sector stressed the importance of using spare capacity in private hospitals, particularly during the winter months. The recent election manifestos of both the Labour Party and the Conservative Party also outlined plans for the private sector to manage specially built surgical units for non-emergency operations.

Policies which enable more flexible access to services form another important element of the strategy to reduce waiting times. Initiatives introduced by the current Government include NHS Direct, a telephone service providing health information and advice, and walk-in primary care centres, both of which are nurse led and available 24 hours a day. These services seek to ensure the NHS delivers more convenient, patient-centred care that meets the needs of modern lifestyles. They have been influenced by wider developments in society where people can increasingly access services throughout the day and night, such as on-line banking.

A range of other policies are being implemented to deliver care as quickly and conveniently as possible, and to ensure that services are designed around the needs of patients rather than the needs of professionals or the system as a whole. For example, new collaborative programmes are reducing the number of appointments and hospital visits required for tests and results to help cut waiting times and reduce patient anxiety. Other patient-centred initiatives include improving hospital menus and the cleanliness of wards, booked appointments systems (due to be delivered across the NHS by 2005) and installing bedside televisions and telephones.

A 'primary-care led' NHS

The overall direction of health policy is towards delivering a 'primary-care led' health service. The Conservative Government's GP Fundholding scheme and the current administration's Primary Care Groups and Trusts have all helped devolve responsibility for commissioning and providing services to the local level. The focus on primary care is set to increase over the coming years. The Government has made much of its plans to devolve more power and resources to 'front line staff'. Changes in health professionals roles (see below) will also contribute to this trend. For example, the NHS Plan proposes new specialist GPs in ophthalmology, orthopaedics, dermatology, and ear nose and throat surgery to improve the availability of these services at the local level.

Moves to improve the integration between health and social care are relevant here. Governments of all political persuasions have attempted to bridge divides between health and social care, which have long been a source of confusion to patients and frustration to professionals. Recent initiatives include a series of measures passed in the 1999 Health Act to enable the NHS and local councils to work more closely together, such as pooled budgets, lead commissioning (where either the NHS or local government can commission services on behalf of both organisations), and merging local and health authority services into one-stop packages of care. The current Government aims to increase the pace of change in this area, particularly in relation to services for older people. New intermediate care services are being encouraged, including rapid response teams to provide emergency care for people at home and prevent unnecessary hospital admissions, intensive rehabilitation services to help older patients regain their health and independence after a stroke or major surgery, and integrated home care teams to ensure that people receive the care they need when they are discharged from hospital. In future, Care Trusts (a new level of Primary Care Trust) will be responsible for commissioning and providing all health and social care at the local level.

Whilst the overall policy emphasis is on delivering healthcare closer to people's homes, certain services – for example Accident and Emergency and cancer services – are becoming increasingly specialised as part of the drive to improve standards and produce better patient outcomes. A key theme highlighted by the Calman Hine report is that the future organisation and delivery of services will focus on co-ordinated networks of care which will manage conditions across services, rather than services based around existing structures and buildings. The objective is to ensure services are delivered at the most appropriate level according to the best available clinical evidence, and a series of National Service Frameworks have outlined how this should be achieved in practice. A vision of how services might be provided in f[illegible] is provided by the results of the National Beds Inquiry:

> Knowledge is likely to be centralised in the hospital but services will be spun out to the periphery. Telemedicine is expected to enhance this process. Some see the major acute hospital of the future as a resource centre for high technology, high cost, high risk interventions. It would operate as a hub from which expertise and advice is available to wider health networks including a range of local facilities dealing with less risky and/or severe conditions, for example ambulatory care centres, minor injury units and rehabilitation units (Department of Health 2000b).

Changes in health professionals' roles

Although there have been a number of changes to different health professionals roles over recent years, the current Government has particularly emphasised this trend. The NHS Plan makes a number of proposals to 'break down the barriers between NHS staff'. These primarily focus on expanding the role of nurses, for example through the new walk-in centres and NHS Direct and through increased responsibilities for prescribing. Wider roles for other health professionals, including pharmacists, health visitors and midwives, are also envisaged (Department of Health, 2000a).

These developments are taking place for a number of reasons. They are in part to help cut waiting times by reducing GPs' and other doctors' workloads. They are also a response to demands from health professionals themselves to more fully develop their skills and potential within the NHS. Evolving professional roles are also being driven by outside forces. It has been suggested that in some deprived parts of the country up to a quarter of GPs will soon be lost, mainly due to the impending retirement of Asian GPs. The potential for nurse-led services has already been highlighted as a feasible alternative in these areas (Taylor and Esmail, 1999).

Changes in patients' roles

The patient's role in healthcare is also changing. As already o[illegible]ed, patients are becoming more informed and less deferential. Ho[illegible] need to improve both the quality and quantity of information available to patients is increasingly being recognised. The Centre for Health Information Quality was set up by the Government in 1997 to help raise standards in the production of health information and NHS Direct Online is helping patients to access good quality information on the web. A Cancer Information Advisory Group has been established to improve the quality of information for cancer patients. The National Electronic Library for Health will also include cancer information specifically for patients (Sowden and Forbes, 2001).

Information on how the NHS as a whole is performing is also being developed. The Department of Health first published its High Level Performance Indicators and Clinical Indicators for Health Authorities and Trusts two years ago, and last year the indicators were brought together into a single publication in order to improve accessibility.[10] These indicators are based on the NHS's new Performance Assessment Framework which covers six key areas: health improvement (including death and accident rates), fair access (waiting times for certain conditions and treatments), the effective delivery of appropriate healthcare (such as rates for childhood immunisation and returning home following treatment for a stroke), efficiency (including length of stay and levels of generic prescribing), the patient/carer experience of the NHS (for example the number of cancelled operations or delayed discharge) and health outcomes (including conceptions below age 18, infant mortality rates, survival rates for different cancers and deaths in hospital following surgery).

Whilst the publication of these indicators has been welcomed, they have also been criticised for being insufficiently patient friendly. Non-official sources are beginning to emerge from outside Government. The King's Fund health charity is currently seeking to translate the Performance Indicators for London into a more accessible format that patients can access via the internet. The College of Health's waiting list help line can provide patients with waiting lists for individual consultants. The *Sunday Times* recently produced its own version of hospital league tables. These tables included information relating hospital mortality rates to the number of doctors, and data from 'Dr Foster', a private company which collects and publishes data on individual hospitals on the web. Dr Foster's league tables include information on the general services each hospital provides, the quality of care available (assessed according to issues like the number of doctors and nurses per bed and general inpatient and outpatient waiting times), and information on how to get to the hospital and whether or not it has a newsagent or gift shop.[11] These developments and are likely to keep the pressure on Government to make its own information more patient friendly in future.

Policies are also being developed to enable patients to become more involved in their own healthcare. Patients groups have long recognised that people living with long-term and chronic conditions may be more knowledgeable about their own condition than health professionals. As the UK population ages, the number of people living with a long-term condition is set to increase. It has been argued that medical interventions alone will be insufficient to meet the challenges this trend raises and that self-management programmes are an additional resource that should be used to add value to existing healthcare provision and to support people to become more efficient users of health and social services. More importantly, there is evidence which suggests that self-management interventions can have a beneficial impact on health (Cooper 2001). In response to these issues, the Government has established an Expert Patient programme to explore how patients with long term and chronic conditions could be more effectively supported in future.[12] The Long-Term Medical Conditions Alliance has recently published the results of its Living with Long-term Illness (or Lill) Project to feed into the Expert Patient programme. It found that after just four months of attending self-management courses, participants gained statistically significant improvements in self-efficacy, use of self management techniques, health status and healthcare utilisation (Cooper, 2001).

Another policy area where the importance of the patients' role has been recognised by Government, health professionals and industry is in medicines taking. It is likely that medicines will become more easily available in future as pharmacy medicines, instead of prescription only medicines, and as general sale list medicines instead of pharmacy medicines. This could enable greater opportunities for self-care amongst a broad range of patients. It has been argued that the key factors promoting the reclassification of drugs include patient empowerment, the rise of consumerism, the changing balance of power between health professionals, pharmacists' drive to extend their role, Government policy to contain the NHS drugs bill, pharmaceutical companies' desire to increase their profits and the possible influence of healthcare systems outside Britain (Blenkinsopp and Bradley, 1996). A Joint Task Force involving Government, the professions, the pharmaceutical industry and patient groups has recently been established to implement a national strategy on partnership in medicine taking. The strategy seeks to promote a 'concordance' approach in medicine taking. This approach recognises that patients are not simply passive recipients of prescribing decisions but also have their own beliefs about medicines, how they work and how they are best used. It has been suggested that the concordance concept could help to reduce avoidable ill health, admissions to hospitals, the proportion of wasted medicines and even premature death, as well as increase patient satisfaction.[13] Key issues the strategy will seek to address include improving the education and training of health professionals in the concordance approach, raising public awareness and spreading best practice (Department of Health, 2000c).

It has been argued that we need to move beyond simply encouraging patients to become more informed and to take on new responsibilities for medication. Support for the 'shared decision-making' model has grown in recent years.[14] This is intended to be a genuinely partnership approach to healthcare and could lead to significant improvements in health. There is evidence, for example, that patients with hypertension benefit if they are allowed to adopt an active rather than a passive role in treatment, patients with breast cancer suffer less depression and anxiety if they are treated by doctors who adopt a participative consultation style, and patients who are more actively involved in discussion about the management of their diabetes achieve better blood sugar control (Coulter *at al*, 1999).

A final point in relation to changing patient roles is the current and likely future policy emphasis on ensuring the voice of patients and the public is heard more widely in the health service. Commentators have long criticised the 'democratic deficit' in the NHS and argued that involving patients and the wider public in decisions about how services are run is vital to improving the quality of care provided and because of wider accountability issues (Cooper *et al*, 1995). The current Government proposes to establish a new Patient Advocacy and Liaison Service, Independent Local Advisory Forums of local people to provide

ɔ patients want from their health
ɔs?

The secon section of this report assesses the likely wants, needs and expectations of future patients, outlining issues including where patients are likely to want to be treated, how they will want to access care and who they might want to be treated by.

It is important to begin by understanding what patients generally want from the health service and the staff who work in it. The three key issues that come up time and time again are that patients want quicker, more flexible access to treatment, they want good quality relationships with health professionals, and they want to be more informed.

Quicker, more flexible access

There is considerable evidence that the public's top concern about the NHS is waiting for treatment. The National Survey of NHS Patients indicates that the highest levels of patient discontent are about accessing GP services and waiting times for hospital appointments and treatment. Groups who seem particularly dissatisfied include people under 45 years old, those living in London (partly because the capital has a young population) and people from ethnic minority groups. Those in paid work and in full time education are the least satisfied with arrangements for accessing their GP surgery. Interestingly, the National Survey reveals few social class differences in this respect (Department of Health, 1998).

Qualitative research confirms that waiting times are a key priority for patients. By far the most frustrating experience of the NHS is that of waiting: waiting for a doctor's appointment, waiting for an appointment with a specialist or consultant, waiting in the doctor's surgery or hospital once you have an appointment, waiting to be discharged, waiting to be seen in casualty and so on. There is some evidence that older patients face particular problems, such as being put at the bottom of waiting lists or even being denied treatment altogether, specifically because of their age (Gilchrist, 1999). For the patient, waiting means not being in control, getting anxious, wasting time and generally feeling unimportant (Edwards, 2001). People feel the issue of waiting needs to be resolved before other important issues facing the NHS can be ldressed (Lenaghan, 1999). The main reason why people are style, where the doctor specifically leads communication and seeks to diagnose the patients' problem through text book style enquiries about the symptoms and medical history. There have been extensive studies investigating the relationship between 'patient-centredness' in doctors and patients' satisfaction with the care they receive. These studies have found that patients are more likely to be satisfied when their doctors' behaviour is facilitating rather than dominating. Higher patient satisfaction has also been associated with higher use of patient-centred communications (giving information and counselling) and lower use of doctor-centred communication (giving directions and asking questions) (Williams and Calnan, 1991). However, a major barrier to achieving patient-centred, individualised care is the lack of time available during consultations (Williams *et al*, 1998).

The interpersonal skills of healthcare professionals have been found to be of paramount importance in determining the extent to which patients are satisfied with the care they receive (Walker *et al*, 1998). Patients are more likely to be satisfied with the consultation if the doctor's manner is friendly rather than business like, and where the doctor engages in social, non-medical conversation. Unsurprisingly, consultations where there is a negative tone – anger, tension or antagonism either from the patient or the doctor – are associated with dissatisfaction. Encouraging and empathic behaviours of physicians towards patients have been found to be have a positive impact on patients' attitudes whilst doctors' perceived failure to take problems seriously has been found to have a negative impact. Overall, patients' liking of the doctor as a person and having faith in them is a key factor in determining whether or not patients are satisfied with the care and treatment they receive (Williams and Calnan, 1991).

So the available evidence points to a range of factors being important to patients in terms of the care they receive – not just how long they have to wait or how easily they can access services, important though these issues are – and that patients' relationships with health professionals are at the heart of the issue. It is important to note that there are significant differences in how different groups of patients feel they are treated by health professionals. For example, the National Survey of NHS Patients provides some interesting evidence about patients' perceptions of GPs. Women are more likely than men to be critical of GPs' behaviour towards them. They are more likely to say that

GPs do not provide them with enough information and that there tends to be insufficient time during consultations to ask questions. Younger people are less likely to think GPs spend enough time with them than older groups. Women aged under 25 years tend to be the most critical group. They are much less likely than older patients to agree that GPs always listen to them, take their views seriously or treat them with courtesy and respect (Department of Health, 1998).

People from ethnic minority groups also tend to take a less favourable view of their treatment by GPs, although these differences are smaller if the younger age profile of this group is taken into account. Ethnic groups are more doubtful about their GP making the right diagnosis and knowing which treatment is best for them and consequently more likely to want a second opinion. People from ethnic minorities are less likely to say their GP always treats them with courtesy and respect and listens to them. They are twice as likely as white respondents to say their GP does not given them enough information about their treatment or condition. The state of a person's health is another important predictor of patient satisfaction. The worse a person's health, the more critical they are likely to be of their GP's willingness or ability to answer questions and the more likely they are to feel unable to both ask questions or understand the answers (Department of Health, 1998).

High quality, timely information

Patients generally feel very ill informed in today's NHS. This lack of information is apparent at every level of the patient's experience: from not knowing what is going to happen to them when they go into hospital and how long their treatment will take, to a lack of information about the purpose and potential effects of medicines they are taking. Finding out what is often very basic information is one of the main 'battles' patients struggle to cope with in their contact with the health service. The type of information that patients want is varied and covers both general information about the quality of the service as a whole – such as waiting list times, success rates for particular operations and the qualifications and credentials of individual professionals – and information relevant to the individual patient, including what the treatment or operation will entail, who is going to perform it, how long the process will take, what the recovery rate is, what if any medicine will be required and any potential side effects (Edwards, 2001). Even when patients do receive information it often fails to meet their needs. Research suggests that patients want to have as much information about the possible side effects of treatments as possible, so long as it is presented in a non-alarmist manner. This is contrary to the assumptions of many information providers and is therefore often missing from patient information (Coulter *et al*, 1999).

Whilst many patients clearly feel ill informed, they are also fearful about the consequences of opening up the NHS to greater public scrutiny. Developments like league tables could challenge patients' beliefs or hopes that the health service is infallible, that doctor's do not make mistakes, that all health professionals or hospitals are as good as one another and so on. Highlighting the weaknesses of the service may simply serve to frighten some patients and make them feel even less confident and in control, rather than to empower them. In general, patients find it very difficult to imagine a situation where they would have a choice in deciding the course and location of treatment they wish to pursue (Edwards, 2001).

Where do patients want to be treated?

This paper has already suggested that both the future health policy agenda and the onset of new technologies like telemedicine are likely to increase the amount of services provided at the local level. Patients are likely to welcome this trend. Patients want to be treated as close to where they live as possible and support moves to provide more services in their local community rather than in acute hospital settings. Familiar surroundings and proximity to family members and friends are key factors here. Patients seem particularly attracted by the idea of spending more time after treatment at home, so long as health professionals can visit them to ensure there aren't any problems (Lenaghan, 1999).

Developments which enable more care to be delivered locally, like outreach clinics and telemedicine, are likely to be welcomed by patients. A recent study evaluating the costs and effectiveness of specialist outreach clinics in general practice, for example, found that patients who used the clinics were more satisfied than those who went to the more traditional hospital outpatient clinic. A number of factors contributed to this satisfaction, including the length of time to get an appointment to see the specialist, the convenience of location of the outreach clinic, the length of time spent waiting to see the specialist at the clinic, the time spent with the specialist at the clinic, the convenience of the day and time of the appointment, the waiting area and the attention that was given to what the patient had to say during the consultation. Three quarters of the patients who used the outreach clinics said they preferred to be treated at the GP's surgery rather than going to hospital. Only one in five of the patients seen in the hospital outpatient clinic said they preferred to be seen in the hospital: 44 per cent said they would have preferred to have been seen in the GP's surgery (Bowling *et al* 1997).

A systematic review of patient satisfaction with teleconsultations with specialists using real time interactive videos found that patients see distinct advantages to teleconsultation, particularly the availability of specialist services at the local level, the fact that less travel is required and that waiting times are reduced.[16] (Mair and Whitten, 2000) Qualitative research supports this analysis:

> *If it's saving time and money then yeah, it's a good thing.*
>
> *On TV there was an old lady in his surgery and he used a computer to take an image and it was then sent through to a specialist who diagnosed her. She was seen within a week.*
>
> (Edwards, 2001)

It is important that the potential for 'trade-offs' is considered when looking at where patients might prefer to be treated now and in the future. If patients want to see the 'best' doctor for their particular condition, they may have to wait longer or travel further. Different groups of patients may react differently to such trade-offs. This issue was explored in recent qualitative research conducted by IPPR. The prospect of travelling for treatment is considered worthwhile in order to receive treatment more quickly. In an ideal world patients would be able to access all healthcare services closer to home but most patients are reconciled with the fact that this is not how the NHS works. Patients are quick to make the trade-off between travelling further and receiving prompt treatment, therefore reducing pain and anxiety; '*If you had a bad hip and three hours travel would save you six months of pain, you would definitely do it.*' However, such willingness to travel tends not to extend to older patients or to emergency treatment (Edwards, 2001).

How do patients want to access services?

The traditional method of accessing health services – through face to face consultations in the local GP's surgery – is already changing. NHS Direct enables people to get advice and information on the telephone and walk in centres are providing access 24 hours a day. New technologies are likely to provide new opportunities for accessing services in future.

Using the telephone and email

Patients' attitudes towards using the telephone to access health services can be assessed by looking at their views about NHS Direct. The vast majority of people who use NHS Direct appear to be satisfied with the service they receive and are quick to recommend it to others. Patients particularly value the reassurance and advice the service provides. Patients who use NHS Direct are predominantly parents. Research indicates that many men, ethnic minorities and younger age groups are unaware that the service exists. This suggests that the service should be advertised and promoted more widely to increase access amongst these groups (Edwards, 2001). It is important to be aware that there may be some wariness amongst patients about the possibility of greater use of the telephone in future. These concerns are important because the use of the telephone is set to expand over the coming years.[17] Whilst patients can envisage using the telephone for more basic needs such as minor ailments, repeat prescriptions and straightforward advice and information, the possibility of using the telephone for more complex consultations may not be welcomed. Many patients feel they would be unable to describe their symptoms accurately or effectively over the phone (Edwards, 2001).

Patients' attitudes towards the potential use of email are similar to that of the telephone. On the plus side, patients can envisage using email to find out extra information after a consultation has taken place, for example on medicines that have been prescribed, or to get a second opinion. However, views about more interactive use of email are more negative. Patients feel that accurately writing down symptoms in an email would be even more problematic than describing them over the phone:

> *You can speak faster than you can write can't you? I would rather speak to someone...you can gauge the sort of person you are talking to by the way they talk back to you.*
> (Edwards, 2001)

Patients also worry that 'big' medical terms in written response would be difficult to understand and that the system could be open to abuse, for example it could be difficult to check professionals' credentials.

Impact of new technologies on professional patient relationship

Some patients think new technologies could help improve the professional patient relationship. Qualitative research suggests that patients may welcome the use of telemedicine because it will help professionals share knowledge and information around the world, thereby increasing the chance of finding a solution:

> *I went to one specialist and he sort of photographed whatever and sent it off round the world to get other views on it. People from around the world then came back, they obviously accessed his website and he used the information.*
> (Edwards, 2001)

However, most patients are concerned that using new technologies to access services could harm the professional patient relationship and reduce the 'personal touch' which they so value. An evaluation of telepsychiatry in the North West of England, for example, found that whilst patients were not fazed by the technology *per se*, they were concerned that it might prevent genuinely full and frank communication between doctor and patient. Patients were worried that the psychiatrist might not understand what they meant if he could not see their faces clearly (May *et al*, 2000).

Older patients appear particularly wedded to face-to-face consultations, seeing them as critical in securing accurate diagnoses. Patients also think privacy is very important: '*Your body is very personal and you want somebody who you can trust and who you think is a bit personal.*' Younger respondents fear that televisual images could be subject to abuse and too easily accessed by others around the world: '*It could get abused, seriously abused. You may have a rash on your bottom or something and the next thing you know, it's on the internet!*'. However, patients who have seen demonstrations of telemedicine, either on television or in person, may be more positive about it suggesting that it is unfamiliarity and lack of knowledge rather than a deeper opposition that makes patients sceptical about the use of telemedicine in future (Edwards, 2001).

Continuity of care

GPs have traditionally been the foundation of the UK's system of healthcare, playing a key role in ensuring there is continuity of care. Some family doctors argue that retaining the direct link between GPs and their patients is vital, in part because knowing an individual patient's medical history helps improve diagnosis and treatment outcomes but also because this is 'what patients want'. Others refute this argument. They suggest that not all patients regard having a continual relationship with the same GP as important and question whether GPs retaining control over the medical records of their patients is as central to health outcomes or continuity of care as was once thought (Mihill, 2000).

What do patients think about these issues? The National Survey of NHS Patients suggests that less than 50 per cent of patients think their GP knows 'a lot' about their medical history. Around a third say their GP knows 'a fair amount' and 16 per cent say their GP knows little or nothing. When questioned specifically about their last visit to their GP, patients express relatively little concern about the level of their GP's knowledge, with eight out of ten patients saying their GP knew enough (Department of Health, 1998).

There is evidence that the doctor-patient tie is less sacrosanct than it is often held up to be, particularly among younger age groups. Many patients, particularly younger patients and men, say that in most situations they would be happy to see any doctor. Patients might prefer to see their usual doctor but in the majority of cases being seen quickly is more of a priority. This is particularly true for minor conditions, repeat prescriptions and recurring symptoms. Furthermore, patients recognise that accessing different doctors could be beneficial since it would expose them to 'different ways of doing things' and thereby help promote greater choice. In this sense the traditional doctor patient relationship model can be seen as limiting and may result in patients feeling they are 'stuck' with a particular doctor with little sense of what alternatives might be available (Edwards, 2001). However, having the same GP is far more important for some patients, such as older patients and those with on-going or serious conditions. Patients often want the reassurance of speaking to someone who understands and empathises with their condition and who knows their history of dealing with it:

> *If I'm only going for HRT replacement I see anybody, but if I'm going for something ongoing then I see what I call my doctor which is the one I'm registered with.*
> (Edwards, 2001).

Furthermore, whilst patients do not feel tied to seeing the same doctor in every appointment, many do seem to value the familiarity of their local surgery or health centre. Some patients seem to associate walk-in-centres with services for homeless people or drug users and on this basis assume that they could be run-down or poor quality. Patients also say they need reassurance about the experience and qualifications of the health professionals working in such centres. However, these views may be due to a lack of experience or familiarity with the service rather than a problem with the concept of 'off-the-street' services *per se*. An interesting point is that negative responses to walk-in-centres appear more pronounced among women than men (Edwards, 2001).

Who do patients want to be treated by?

Relatively little attention has so far been given to patients' views towards the trend towards 'breaking down barriers' between NHS staff (Chapple *et al*, 2000). Yet understanding public attitudes about professionals like nurses and pharmacists will be vital if proposals to break down staff barriers are to be accepted and effectively implemented, both now and in the future.

Nurses

Nurses have taken on increased responsibilities for healthcare over recent years and this trend is set to continue in future. Nurses are leading new services like NHS Direct and walk-in-centres. Other developments include nurse-led triage in Accident and Emergency departments, nurse prescribers and nurse consultants.

The evidence about public perceptions of nurses' current roles appears very favourable. According to the National Survey of NHS Patients, nurses are seen as being more likely to take appropriate action, more likely to answer questions and more likely to be easily understood than GPs (Department of Health, 1998). In general, patients seem to feel that making more use of nurses is beneficial, both to patients – because nurses are seen to have the personal touch that GPs are thought to lack – and to GPs, helping to reduce their workload and save money. Patients have already noticed nurses taking on more responsibility in local health centres, for example giving 'flu jabs, taking blood pressure and so on. Most are comfortable with these developments and some wish nurses roles could be expanded further still:

> *It's a shame they [nurses] can't prescribe because I think some of them are so well qualified that they know exactly what's wrong because they see people all the time.*
> (Edwards, 2001).

However, these views are not universally held. Some older people feel that GPs may be pushing people to see the nurse simply to relieve their own workloads, rather than because it is beneficial to patients (IPPR, 1998). Patients stress that nurses should not become a barrier between patients and the doctor: patients want to be able to choose to see their doctor if they prefer. Older people are particularly likely to want to see their GP rather than the nurse. In contrast, young and middle class patients feel that nurses have more time and better qualifications than in the past. Patients are also concerned not to over-burden nurses and that they should be properly rewarded for any increase in responsibilities (Edwards, 2001).

A recent study of a nurse led Personal Medical Services pilot scheme in Salford suggests that patients' attitudes towards nurses must be seen in the context of the history of the service and wider socio-cultural attitudes such as perceived gender roles. The study showed that patients both accepted and welcomed an expanded role for nurses. The social support and continuity of care provided by the nurse was a key factor in the high levels of satisfaction and confidence expressed by patients. Patients saw the nurse as highly qualified, competent and knowledgeable. Some patients spoke of the nurse as though he were a doctor. Patients particularly appreciated the time the nurse spent with them and the fact that he seemed very approachable and at ease with them. However, patients' attitudes may have been influenced by previous dissatisfaction with the service they were receiving. In the period immediately prior to the nurse-led scheme starting, the practice had been run by a series of locums and other doctors which many patients had been unhappy with. This was in stark contrast to what most patients had been used to, since the practice had previously been run by a single GP for twenty-five years. The nurse's gender is also an issue for consideration. The fact that the nurse who led the practice in Salford was a man does not appear to have been an important factor in how patients perceived his role. However, the authors of the study say they cannot be sure that a female nurse would have commanded the same level of support from all patients in all cultures (Chapple *et al*, 2000).

Pharmacists

Current and future trends in health policy are likely to increase pharmacists' roles and responsibilities. Relevant developments include new Electronic Health Records which could enable pharmacists to issue repeat prescriptions, promoting the concept of 'concordance' approach to medicine taking and the increasing availability of medicines 'over the counter'. The NHS Plan suggests that a key factor determining pharmacists' future roles will be the shift away from paying pharmacists mainly for the dispensing of individual prescriptions towards rewarding overall service. Personal Medical Services type schemes are set to pilot alternative contracts for pharmacy services, covering issues like medicines management and repeat prescribing (Department of Health, 2000a).

Research suggests patients think pharmacists have improved over recent years. They are no longer seen as 'shop keepers' and instead are regarded as an important member of the primary healthcare team (IPPR, 1998). Many patients hold pharmacists in high esteem and see them as being extremely knowledgeable, particularly in relation to minor ailments and conditions. The training and qualifications necessary to become a pharmacist are recognised by many patients. Patients are already noticing developments in how local pharmacists work, such as computer records of patients' previous prescriptions. Furthermore, some patients say they would be happy for pharmacists to prescribe medicines for patients (albeit within proper guidelines) or to give patients' repeat prescriptions without having to refer them back to the GP (Edwards, 2001).

Many pharmacy users act as proxy consulters, asking for information for friends and relatives. Women in particular seem to use the pharmacy on behalf of their children. People may also use the pharmacy as a 'stepping stone' to see their GP (in other words they visit the pharmacist to ascertain whether their condition is serious enough to warrant a visit to the GP). However, people also use their pharmacy for more negative reasons: for example, because they find it difficult to get an appointment with their GP or because they are afraid of being ridiculed or fobbed off by the doctor (Hassell *et al*, 1997).

In general, patients appear happy with the notion of increasing the responsibilities of health professionals like nurses and pharmacists so long as it is matched with more training. This attitude is partly a result of a sort of 'blind faith' in health professionals, an attitude that '*if they are doing the job then they must be able and qualified to do it*'. However, this attitude could change if trust in health professionals declines in the wake of recent scandals about criminal or negligent doctors and nurses. Furthermore, patients currently support changing professional roles because they want to be given more time in the NHS. Time is a precious and rare commodity in the health service and patients believe that nurses and pharmacists tend to have more time to spend talking through patients' concerns and queries (Edwards, 2001). Again, these attitudes could change in future if increased workloads for nurses and pharmacists reduce the amount of time they can spend with patients.

Complementary and alternative practitioners

Another issue which may be relevant in terms of who delivers healthcare in future is the potential role of complementary and alternative practitioners. A significant proportion of people in the UK currently use complementary or alternative medicines (CAM) and it is predicted that this proportion will increase in future (Pahl, 1999). It has been suggested that every week, around 40 per cent of GPs recommend or endorse the use of CAM and one in five refers their patients to these services. Surveys in countries like Norway, New Zealand and the Netherlands, show similar results (Paterson and Britten, 1999).

People use CAM because of positive reasons – they are seen as being more patient-centred and holistic – and because of negative perceptions of orthodox treatment, which may be seen as ineffective and having unknown or adverse side-effects. Paterson and Britten found that whilst some people who use complementary therapy say they are hoping to find a 'cure', most simply want to establish a degree of control over their situation and be able to cope better with their illness:

> *It is ridiculous to just go on...you've got to take some action and I'm learning to do that.*
>
> *I wasn't expecting a miracle cure, but I thought that he would help me just get a bit better and to help myself...to carry on.*
>
> (Paterson and Britten, 1999)

People who use CAM tend to be well educated: one study found the majority of users were educated to degree level (Vincent and Furnham, 1996). Interestingly, some research suggests that a significant proportion of those who use alternative or complementary therapies are health professionals (Paterson and Britten, 1999). European studies have shown that women are more likely to take herbal or homeopathic remedies than men (Pahl, 1999). This finding is supported by a recent survey of users of over the counter (OTC) homeopathic medicines which found that around 80 per cent were women. The survey also found that people who used OTC homeopathic medicines tend to be older people with chronic conditions: only five per cent of users were aged under 25 years old. This finding supports the suggestion that the use of alternative and complementary therapies may increase in future as the population ages and more people live with chronic conditions (Paterson and Britten, 1999).

The trend towards increasing use of complementary or alternative medicines raises a number of challenges for government, alternative practitioners and conventional health professionals. These include improving the evidence base of CAM, ensuring there is an independent source of information for both patients and conventional health professionals on what works and what does not, improving the regulation of certain CAM practitioners, and improving the awareness of CAM amongst conventional practitioners (House of Lords, 2000).

Qualitative research suggests that patients would welcome the integration of complimentary and alternative medicines more fully into the UK's system of healthcare as a 'common sense' approach, so long as treatments are backed by research which supports their effectiveness. Some patients want to see alternative medicines and treatments becoming part and parcel of what the NHS does for pragmatic reasons: '*if it works, why not give it a go?*'. Others are enthusiasts and value the concept of more natural, less intrusive approaches to healthcare: '*Doctors will pump you full of drugs as opposed to referring you on to something else.*' For many patients the issue is essentially one of choice: '*Doctors should be aware of this and they should also be trained about different choices that you have.*' However, patients do not always see alternative medicine in a positive light. Concern is expressed over bogus practitioners and patients can be sceptical about the benefits CAM might bring. Part of this scepticism may be a result of a feeling that doctors do not always subscribe to the value of alternative medicines and if they do, it is often as a last resort. While some patients have tried alternative medicines on the advice of their doctor, others have taken a more hit and miss approach. Beyond looking for qualifications from an authoritative body, patients have little notion of how else they might be reassured by the credentials of alternative practitioners. There are indications that patients would welcome more information about what alternatives are available and clearer guidelines on the best people to go to (Edwards, 2001).

What do patients want to be treated for?

The answer to the above question may seem obvious. However the next five to fifteen years could bring developments that enable patients to be treated for diseases or conditions which they regard as quite different from those the NHS currently seeks to address. Two issues serve to illustrate this point. Firstly, there may be an increase in so-called lifestyle drugs that treat conditions which may not necessarily be considered to constitute 'ill health'. Secondly, developments emerging from the human genome project, including genetic tests to predict the future onset of disease and gene therapy to replace faulty genes, may be seen to fundamentally change what patients and the wider public are 'treated' for in future.

Lifestyle drugs

Do patients and the wider public think that the conditions which lifestyle drugs 'treat' – such as baldness, obesity and impotence – constitute ill health? If not, do patients think they should be available on the NHS? IPPR has previously conducted qualitative research on this issue. When asked to consider where responsibility for different lifestyle drugs should lie, people gave the following responses. Broadly speaking, Propecia (a drug to tackle baldness) was seen as predominantly a matter of personal responsibility, eliciting comments such as: '*Baldness is not an illness.*' and '*The NHS has more important things to spend its money on.*' Viagra (a drug to combat the symptoms of erectile dysfunction) was considered to be 'down the middle'. Attitudes towards where responsibility should lie are best summed up by the comment '*If you have a real problem you should get a prescription, but if you just want more sex you should pay for it.*' Xenical (a drug to tackle weight problems such as obesity) was seen as largely a matter for the NHS: '*It's life threatening if you are obese*', although concern was expressed about the possibility of abuse: '*You would have 14 or 15 year old girls abusing it.*' (New, 2000).

So patients understand that the NHS cannot, and indeed should not necessarily provide every treatment that is available. People appear most comfortable with restricting treatments which are (potentially) for cosmetic purposes and therefore not considered a health issue. Patients do not want to be prevented from accessing these treatments; they simply recognise that some lifestyle drugs should be considered the individual's responsibility and paid for as such.

Genetics

Public ideas about genetics in general appear to be very loosely formed at present. A lack of information and knowledge about genetics means that many people see it as a frightening, complicated and even meddlesome area of expertise: one which 'messes with nature' in a profound way (Edwards, 2001). A recent MORI survey looked at public attitudes towards the use of genetic information[18]. It found that whilst nine out of ten people agreed that genetic developments could and should be used to diagnose and bring about cures for diseases in future, one third were concerned that research on human genetics was tampering with nature and therefore unethical. Women were more likely than men to think that the new genetics is tampering with nature, by 37 per cent to 28 per cent. Furthermore, three quarters of people felt they had little information about the controls on biological developments and most had little or no confidence that rules and regulations were keeping pace with new scientific developments. Young people were more likely to lack confidence in controls than older people. Unsurprisingly, respondents with a high level of knowledge about genetics were more likely to be positive about the potential health benefits than those with low levels of knowledge.

If patients' attitudes towards genetics in general are sceptical, their attitudes towards genetic testing in particular are even more negative. It has been argued that patients' views about genetic testing are likely to depend upon a complex combination of factors, including public knowledge and perception of genetics in general and of each disease and test in particular. In addition, potential public demand for genetic tests must be viewed in the context of a wider cultural shift towards more self-medication and patient autonomy (Lenaghan, 1998). (Patients' attitudes towards self-care are discussed in further detail below.) Genetic tests received the most negative response of all the likely future trends in healthcare discussed with patients during IPPR's qualitative research for this paper. A small minority of patients (more likely to be parents, particularly women) were keen to equip themselves with as much knowledge about their and their children's health as possible. (Interestingly the MORI survey also found some evidence that parents of young children may be more likely to hold a positive attitude towards genetics in general, because of the health benefits it could bring.)

However, the majority of people clearly feel that genetic testing is a step too far. Few would contemplate carrying out tests on their own: most would only do so under the close help and guidance of a health professional. Patients were keen that any genetic test would produce unambiguous and easy to interpret results and that they would know exactly what to do with them. This view could prove highly problematic if genetic tests for common, multi-factoral diseases like heart disease and cancer become available. A full understanding of the complex interaction between nature and nurture is still a long way off and genetic tests may only suggest a potential increase in susceptibility. Improving the understanding and communication of risk will therefore become a major challenge in future. Many patients are clearly extremely worried about coping with the results of genetic tests, particularly for serious conditions. Furthermore, the potential benefits of genetic testing (for example encouraging preventive action to be taken) are regarded by some as highly doubtful: '*Someone who smokes and is likely to get cancer is going to know that anyway.*' (Edwards, 2001). People also express a number of concerns about genetic testing in relation to private companies. For example, people are worried that private companies could make profits out of people's fears and uncertainties: '*The people who will make it* [the test] *will make a lot of money because people would generally do it like 2, 3, 4 times just to be sure.*' (Edwards, 2001). The use of genetic information by insurance companies may be a particular cause for concern: MORI found that four out of five people believe that genetic information should not be used by insurance companies, with respondents with a high level of knowledge about genetics being particularly likely to hold this view.

Little research currently exists about patients' attitudes towards individual genetic tests and the evidence that is available indicates that levels of public demand can be difficult to predict accurately. For example, before the test for the single gene disorder Huntington's disease became available, 80 per cent of those with a family history said they would like to know their status. However, once the test became available, only 10 per cent of those with a family history decided to use the test. This can be contrasted with the case of breast cancer. Even though only approximately five per cent of all breast cancers are inherited, there is a high (and arguably inappropriate) level of demand for genetic tests for BRCA1 and BRCA2 (Lenaghan, 1998).

So patients are very concerned about genetics in general and genetic testing in particular. Patients' attitudes about genetics will have major implications for whether and how developments emerging from the human genome project will be implemented in future. There is clearly an urgent need to improve public knowledge in this area and to reassure people about the nature and pace of change. The importance of building public confidence was recognised in a recent speech by the Secretary of State for Health. A number of safeguards to address public concerns have been announced, including support for a moratorium on genetic testing and legislation to ban human reproductive cloning in the UK.[19] Government, professionals, scientists and industry must use the opportunity provided by the Green Paper on genetics, which is due for publication in 2002, to promote wide public debate about the ethical and practical issues raised by the new genetics that dominate patients' concerns.

What role do patients want for themselves?

Perhaps more than in any other area, patient and wider public attitudes towards their future role in healthcare will be critical in determining whether or not potential is turned into reality.

More informed patients?

It is frequently suggested that future patients will be insatiable seekers of information. However, patients' attitudes towards information are often complex: different patients may want different levels of information at different times. Research suggests that patients with particularly severe conditions may be fearful of seeking out additional sources of information. Contradictory information can be a source of anxiety, particularly if treatment decisions have already been made. Self-censorship may occur in order to avoid negative information about illness and preserve hope, which in turn helps patients' manage their fears (Boudioni and McPherson, 2000).

In today's apparently consumer driven era some patients, particularly older patients and men, still prefer not to seek out information. Faith in doctors' expertise still exists and influences patients' information needs. For older patients, this may be because they grew up in a more 'doctor-centred' era. For men, the reason seems to be because they prefer not to ask questions – either of the medical profession or people in their wider social networks – so as to avoid discussion of disease recurrence. Women seem to value the knowledge of other patients in addition to that of health professionals and are therefore more likely to seek information. In contrast, men tend not to rely on the experience of other patients, preferring to try and live life 'as normal'. Men appear to try and retain hope and 'strength in silence'. This has an important effect on their desire for information, particularly through treatment phases (Boudioni and McPherson, 2000).

Indeed, the most noticeably 'information poor' group of patients is men. Men of all ages are consistently less proactive in their information-seeking behaviour. There is an underlying sense that health issues are somehow 'women's issues'. The reasons why seem to differ for younger and older men. Younger men are aware of issues like healthy eating and the importance of fitness. Beyond that, health issues are seen as irrelevant. Young men appear to take pride in the fact that their visits to the doctor are infrequent and look down on those who 'bother' the doctor with 'minor' symptoms. Older men, on the other hand, tend not to seek out health information because they are heavily reliant on others telling them what to do, even if they are suffering from a long term or chronic condition (Edwards, 2001).

However, patients' attitudes towards information may change over time. Younger people see themselves as far more informed than the previous generation and therefore more likely to question their GP. Young people say they get information from a wide variety of sources and that this helps put them in a more powerful position when talking to the GP. Young middle class patients in particular see themselves as the 'information generation'. They are more likely to express concern that GPs are not keeping up with new developments and are subsequently more likely to double check advice. This group tends not to regard the medical profession as the font of all knowledge or as infallible. The media's coverage of recent scandals involving doctors may have had an important affect here. Whilst qualitative research suggests that younger people are generally more critical, young working class people may continue to display residual feelings of deference (IPPR, 1998).

Current sources of information

Whilst the internet is predicted to become a key source of health information in the future, the vast majority of people currently use more traditional sources including health professionals, the media, popular books, newspapers and lay magazines (Rogers *et al*, 1999). An Office of Health Economics' poll found that 48 per cent of people say the most important source of health advice is their GP, 16 per cent say newspapers and magazines, 13 per cent the television, 8 per cent friends and relatives, 6 per cent the practice nurse, health visitor or midwife, 6 per cent the pharmacist and 5 per cent leaflets in the GP's waiting room. Qualitative research supports this analysis. Health professionals are still the first and most trusted source of information although beyond this, patients seek information from a relatively wide range of sources including leaflets from the chemist and friends and family (Edwards, 2001). Gender is an important factor determining the source of health information used. Women are more likely to use magazines, books and the television than men (Illman, 2000). There are also differences in how people from different socio-economic groups access and respond to information. Research suggests that middle class groups are more likely than working class groups to access and respond to health promotion information from leaflets and advertising (Independent Inquiry into Inequalities in Health, 1999). (Gender, age and class differences in the use of health information are returned to below.)

One important source of information currently available to patients is Patient Information Leaflets (PiLs) contained in medicine packs. This is the only information that drug companies are legally required to provide to patients and the only information that patients should be guaranteed to have access to every time they collect a prescription or buy a medicine from a pharmacy. However, research suggests many PiLs do a poor job of helping patients take their medicines safely and effectively. The information contained in many PiLs has been criticised for causing confusion and unnecessary alarm amongst patients. Furthermore, not all patients receive PiLs in their medicines, partly because pharmacists may have to break up pre-packaged medicine to conform to the prescription (Consumers Association, 2000). IPPR's qualitative research supports the view that many patients want more and better information about the medicines they take. Patients feel that medicines which do not contain PiLs make it much harder for them to know what they are taking and why, and packaging for over-the-counter medicines tends to be seen as far more informative (Edwards, 2001).

Patients not only want information about diseases and their treatments, they also want information about the performance of hospitals, health centres and individual professionals. Research suggests that patients would welcome the availability of NHS 'league tables'. Parallels are quickly drawn with school league tables which are seen to enable parents to make more informed choices about their children's education. Patients say that a more robust mechanism for evaluating performance and standards would be better than having to rely solely on the views of family and friends. Patients are very keen that any central source of information should be collected and supplied by an independent body, not the NHS itself, so that it can stand up to proper scrutiny. Patients think that league tables could enable them to make better choices about where they want to be treated and facilitate 'trade-offs', for example if there are shorter waiting lists in other parts of the country some patients would be prepared to travel further afield to get quicker treatment. Patients feel that league tables could also help weed out poorly performing or criminal doctors. However, patients raise concerns about the potential consequences of NHS league tables. Some patients are worried that they could create an even more pressurised environment for health professionals to work in and may not be an effective way of motivating staff already suffering from low morale. Furthermore, knowing where to go to get the 'best treatment' is no guarantee that you will be able to receive that treatment: patients understand that a league table is only truly valuable if it promotes genuine choice. There is concern that being able to evaluate individual health professionals could create pressure and even longer waiting lists for those who are excellent and less work for those with poorer reputations (Edwards, 2001).

Future sources of information

Whilst more traditional sources of information like health professionals and family and friends are currently used to access health information, it is important to consider the potential impact the internet could have since most commentators predict it will play a major role in the future. Qualitative research suggests that very few patients have so far used the internet as a source of health information or advice, although most patients accept that the internet will become far more widely over the coming years. Patients currently see the internet as a tool to collect information rather than as an interactive source of help. Furthermore, it is very much seen as an additional source of information – not a replacement for more traditional sources of advice (Edwards, 2001).

What sort of health information do patients seek on the web? The Health On the Net Foundation (HON), an organisation based in the USA which conducts polls about use of health sites on the web, provides some interesting evidence. Forty six per cent of respondents to a recent HON poll were professionals or students in healthcare, the rest were 'non-medical' users[20]. The majority of 'non-medical' users said they used the internet to look for information on pharmaceutical drugs. Older people were more likely to use the web for this purpose than younger ones. A third of all non-medical respondents said they mostly search the internet for evidence from clinical trials of new pharmaceuticals. Qualitative research in this country seems to support the findings of HON's poll. Patients say they would consider using the internet to find out details on medicines and their potential side effects: '*I think the internet is something for the basics, if you have just got a medicine prescribed or you have just been diagnosed as having an illness you can check it out there*', and information on new or alternative treatments: '*If you had a disease like mine where there's no cure you're constantly looking at new things and the internet is the place you will find them... I just typed in Multiple Sclerosis and it just gave me a lot of references and I tried various sites*' (Edwards, 2001). However, it is important to note that patients do not only search the web for information on the latest drugs and treatment. For example, HON's poll suggests that a substantial proportion of internet users (one third) search for information on patient support groups.

There is considerable evidence that patients are concerned about the reliability of health information available on the web, for example almost three-quarters of non-medical users in HON's poll say the quality of information on the web should be improved. Government policy for addressing this issue is to 'kite-mark' reliable health websites. Whilst there is evidence that patients welcome this initiative (Edwards, 2001) it could be argued that a policy of kite-marking 'approved' sources of information simply reinforces a paternalistic approach to healthcare. Empowering patients with the necessary skills to assess the quality of information they find on the internet would arguably be a more appropriate and modern response.

Who uses health websites in this country? There is little information about the use of health websites according to age, gender, ethnicity or social class. Yet this information will be crucial in developing effective policies to ensure new technologies like the internet do not create a 'digital divide'. Evidence about levels of access amongst different ethnic groups is particularly difficult to come by. Britain is an increasingly multicultural society and likely to become more so in future, but the internet is a predominantly English speaking medium. This could raise important questions about whether and to what extent there are language or cultural barriers in using the internet. Encouraging and enabling equal access amongst different ethnic groups could pose a major challenge to services like NHS Direct Online.

Some information on age and gender related use of health websites can be seen from the HON poll. The poll suggests that women's use of health related websites has grown steadily over recent years and women now make up a clear majority of users. This contrasts with most other types of websites which men are more likely to use. The poll also suggests that North American seekers of on-line health information are older than their European counterparts and far more likely to access the web from home. This is interesting because an internet use first seen in the US often tends to follow here in the UK.

People from disadvantaged groups are far less likely to use the internet as a whole than the wider population.[21] People in social class DE are less likely to have ever used the internet (14 per cent) than the population as a whole (29 per cent). Only 9 per cent of people in social class DE say they have used the internet in the last 12 months, compared with 43 per cent of people in class AB (NOP, 1999). The use oı .. nologies such as the internet and email by benefit recipients is particularly low and there may be a higher resistance to the use of such technologies amongst this group than the population as a whole (Central IT Unit, 1998). Only two per cent of people in social class DE say they have internet access at home, compared with one in three people in social class AB and 14 per cent of all adults (ICM, 1999). This is partly because fewer people in social class DE have a PC at home (25 per cent) compared to the rest of the population (44 per cent) (DTI, 1999). It may also be because in some housing estates, well under half of households have a telephone compared to a national average of over 90 per cent (Social Exclusion Unit, 1999). However, cable and satellite TV ownership is similar amongst DEs (12 per cent and 16 per cent respectively) and ABs (11 per cent and 15 per cent). It has been argued that people may be more likely to extend use of technology which they already understand and feel comfortable with, rather than embarking on something new: 'television is ubiquitous, and digital television may offer a more likely route to home access in [deprived] neighbourhoods in future' (Social Exclusion Unit, 1999).

An increase in self care?

As well as providing new opportunities for patients to become more informed, the future is likely to bring developments which enable patients to take on more responsibilities for their own healthcare. These include programmes which promote greater self-management of diseases and partnerships in medicines taking, the increased availability of medicines available over the counter, and new technologies like home monitoring and diagnostic equipment, telemedicine and even genetic tests. Patients attitudes towards self-care will be crucial in determining if and how these developments are put into practice.

Many patients already take on considerable responsibilities for their own healthcare. One study of over 500 patients found that around half of the illness episodes recorded by the patients during a four week period resulted in self-care activities alone, 17 per cent resulted in self and professional care and five per cent in professional care alone (Rogers *et al*, 1999). Patients claim they understand that effective treatments for minor conditions such as the common cold or 'flu may not be available from their GP. As a result, patients say they tend to wait a few days and try and treat themselves before making a doctor's appointment: '*We will sit and nurse ourselves for two or three days prior to going to the doctor*' although they are more reluctant to wait children are unwell: '*I think most people don't go unless they have to do they? Unless its children. I think with a child you'd rather take him to see a doctor*' (Edwards, 2001).

Yet despite the evidence that many patients already conduct some forms of self-care, patients often fail to see a role for themselves beyond 'doing what they're told': '*I don't know enough about health to say this is the right road. I would rather someone took control and said look, you have this illness, this is what you should do to get yourself better.*' This may be particularly true for older patients who tend to regard moves towards giving patients greater responsibility for their health as about cutting corners and saving money rather than improving patient care (Edwards, 2001).

It may be helpful to look at patients' attitudes towards over the counter medicines (OTCs) as a case study here. Although most research has so far focused on professional attitudes towards the declassification of drugs including general practitioners' desire to protect their domain, pharmacists' anxieties about increasing their own responsibilities, and both professions' doubts about patients' competence in self care (Blenkinsopp and Bradley, 1996) there is some evidence about patients' attitudes that could help illuminate wider debates about the potential for self-care in future. Medicines are generally perceived to be different from other 'supermarket goods' and health professionals, particularly GPs, are seen as an important safety valve. Those who favour OTCs may do so because of negative perceptions of doctors (patients may be afraid or embarrassed about consulting their GP) or because getting repeat prescriptions can be difficult.

Patients are generally concerned about the provision of strong drugs over the counter and the ability of users to administer these drugs wisely. Age and social class factors may be important factors determining attitudes towards OTCs. Young working class patients seem uneasy about the increased availability of OTCs whereas older working class patients seem to like the convenience of being able to pick up drugs from supermarkets. Young middle class patients say they tend not to go to the supermarket to buy drugs, but would pick them up if they were needed although they are also concerned about risks and are doubtful whether people will necessarily read or follow instructions properly. Older middle class people cautiously welcome the increase in OTCs but seem unsure exactly how far the trend should go (IPPR, 1998). Research also points to different attitudes towards OTCs according to ethnicity. A study in Leicester found that Asian patients wanted more information about OTCs than non-Asians, possibly because of the high stress the Asian culture places on education. Overall, Asian patients tend to want fewer medicines available OTC. It has been suggested that this may be because Asians seem to have a higher dependence on doctors than other groups (Rashid *et al*, 1996).

The evidence therefore suggests that whilst a considerable amount of self-care already occurs, many patients do not see a role for themselves beyond doing 'what they are told'. They are reluctant to take on too much responsibility for their own healthcare and instead prefer to rely on health professionals. This may be particularly so for certain groups, such as older patients. However, patients can and do suggest ideas for making self-care easier in future. Younger male patients talk about making access to 'everyday' tests for blood pressure, cholesterol and so on easier, for example by putting them in public places like leisure centres and shopping centres or in the workplace. Other patients say that if medical health checks were a more regular occurrence it would encourage a more preventive approach to health (Edwards, 2001). Wider attitudes towards 'healthy living' may be an important factor in determining whether or not patients are able and willing to take on increased responsibilities for healthcare. There is evidence that an important barrier to people taking on a greater role is that the advice about what is healthy and what is not is constantly changing (IPPR, 1998).

4. The way forward

Patients' views about today's NHS are clear. The vast majority are proud of the health service, particularly the staff who work in it, and want to see it continue in future. But whilst some patients do talk about getting a good standard of care, many are dissatisfied with the treatment they receive. Patients have to wait too long for treatment and even when they are seen, they feel they have to battle to get the time, information and care they need. In this sense, patients' views about what needs to change in future are straightforward. Patients want to spend less time waiting for treatment with more convenient and flexible access to services. They want to spend more time with health professionals so their questions and concerns can be properly addressed. The professional-patient relationship is absolutely central to patients' perceptions of the quality of care they receive.

The next five to fifteen years will bring a vast array of new opportunities to access and deliver health services, through developments like telemedicine, the internet and email. It is important to remember that some patients, particularly older ones, already find the NHS confusing and this confusion could increase as new points of access are added to the system. Many patients are also nervous of these new technologies and the impact they could have on the professional patient relationship. The challenge is therefore be to ensure that different groups of patients can access and use health services in different ways.

A considerable amount is already being done to achieve this goal. NHS Direct and NHS Direct Online are providing health information and advice 24 hours a day, by telephone and online. In some parts of the country, NHS Direct is being taken a step further. In the West Midlands a digital interactive healthcare service is being piloted in 50,000 homes so that patients can get general and local healthcare information, talk to an NHS Direct nurse and even book appointments with the local GP, all on their television screen. A host of other initiatives are taking place to reform health services around the needs of patients, such as the collaborative programmes on cancer and primary care.

The danger is that in rightly seeking to promote greater patient choice, little attention has so far focused on the responsibilities patients might be expected to have in return. A consumerist model of healthcare dominates the current political agenda, as can be seen by the 2001 election manifestos of the three main parties. The Conservatives' manifesto emphasised that they would 'give back to patients and their doctors the power to choose', through a Patient's Guarantee of maximum waiting times that health authorities would be obliged to meet.[22] Labour's manifesto also pledged to 'give patients more choice', by redesigning the NHS around their needs through initiatives like booked appointments and same day tests and diagnosis.[23] The Liberal Democrats' manifesto stressed 'the right to a high quality NHS' proposing a Patient Care Guarantee of minimum standards of treatment.[24] Yet none of these manifestos argued that rights go hand in hand with responsibilities, in sharp contrast to other areas of policy, particularly welfare reform. Providing quicker, more convenient and flexible health services, raising standards of treatment and increasing patient choice are all vital to improving health services in this country. But these moves must go alongside policies which seek to address the other side of equation: the responsibilities or duties patients might be expected to have in return, both as individuals and as members of a wider society.

Establishing a more balanced approach to rights and responsibilities in healthcare will be critical over the coming years. The most important reason why is that empowering individual patients to take on greater responsibility for their own care could help to improve health. Self-management programmes for people with chronic and long-term conditions have demonstrated improved patient outcomes, as well as reducing inappropriate use of services. The concordance or partnership approach to medicine taking could prevent ill health, decrease emergency admissions to hospitals and improve patient satisfaction. The shared decision-making model of healthcare has been shown to reduce patient anxiety and depression and improve health outcomes. The increased availability of over the counter medicines, new home monitoring and diagnostic equipment and telemedicine could all increase the potential for patients to take on more responsibility for their healthcare in future years. Yet the benefits from these developments will be lost if patients are unwilling or unable to take on a greater role.

There are wider reasons why the 'responsibilities' side of the equation must be addressed. Difficult decisions and trade offs between the needs of individual patients and those of the local community and wider society already present a major challenge for policy makers and practitioners. In an increasingly wealthy society, the gap between what patients want and what they get is set to widen further. Information rich patients may find it increasingly difficult to accept the non-availability of a drug or treatment on the NHS if they have access to information proving efficacy in other countries, for example via the internet. Telemedicine could enable UK patients to access and experience health services in other countries, further raising expectations and demand. New technologies, particularly those emerging from the human genome project, are likely to push the costs of healthcare higher still. The new genetics could raise even more profound questions about individual and collective rights and responsibilities. Genetic testing may help identify who is likely to fall ill in future. What responsibilities might society expect these patients to have, for example in taking preventive action? How will more knowledge about who will be ill in future affect wider views about the collective responsibilities for funding and providing care?

If patients are encouraged to view the NHS from a purely consumerist perspective, they will inevitably be dissatisfied and support for the service will be continually undermined. The most advantaged, articulate and wealthy groups in society may decide to opt out of the NHS altogether, leaving the poorest, most vulnerable and disadvantaged patients behind. For those who believe that public services like the NHS play a crucial role in ensuring a fairer, more socially just society this is perhaps the greatest danger of all. The NHS must be transformed to address patients' aspirations for quicker, more flexible and convenient services, but patients must also recognise that the health service is not just another consumer organisations: it is a public service with wider objectives that must be met.

A political choice must therefore be made about the sort of relationship between patients and their health services that should evolve in future: the consumerist model, where the rights of the individual are all powerful, over and above those of the local community or society as a whole, or the citizenship model, where patients have individual rights but also reciprocal responsibilities. This paper argues strongly for the latter approach. Turning this aspiration into reality is one of the most important and difficult health policy challenges to be faced over the coming decades. The scale of the task should not be underestimated. Many patients find it extremely difficult to ask their doctor simple questions about their own illness, let alone share responsibilities for treatment options or take on a degree of responsibility for their care. However, the slow but inevitably decline of paternalism in the NHS provides an important opportunity to drive forward a new agenda: one which genuinely empowers patients by prompting greater choice but also encourages and enables them to take on some responsibilities in return.

Achieving this goal will mean supporting patients to take on new roles as individuals and as members of society at both the local and national level. Exploring how patients should be involved in wider decision-making processes in the NHS has not been the focus of the 'Future Patient' project. The following section therefore explores how individual patients might be enabled to take on new roles and responsibilties. We focus on four key issues: encouraging a more equal professional-patient relationship, providing better information and support for patients and promoting greater patient self-reliance.

A more equal professional-patient relationship

This paper has argued that paternalism, whilst on the decline, still too often dominates health services in this country. Paternalist attitudes are the biggest barrier to patient empowerment and creating more equal relationships between patients and their professionals will be a major challenge over the coming years:

> Assumptions that doctor (or nurse) knows best, making decisions on behalf of patients without involving them and feeling threatened when patients have access to alternative sources of medical information – these signs of paternalism should have no place in a modern system of healthcare. (Coulter, 1999).

As patients become more informed and less deferential, health professionals' roles and responsibilities will need to evolve. Professionals will no longer be the sole providers of knowledge or care. Instead, their role will be to help patients navigate their way through complex and often contradictory information and to assess uncertain risks and benefits (Wyatt, 1998). Professionals' communication skills will become increasingly important and measures are already being taken to ensure these skills are improved. By 2002 it will be a pre-condition of qualification to deliver patient care in the NHS that an individual has demonstrated competence in communication with patients. The communication of risk is likely to become a key issue in the future as new treatments and services emerge from the human genome project. There are tools that health professionals can use to more effectively communicate risk to patients. Presenting information to patients in different ways, for example using descriptive, numerical and graphical formats may be particularly helpful (Edwards *et al*, 1999). However, a more fundamental challenge for health professionals is that they may have to accept that public perceptions of risk are not necessarily 'wrong' but merely different from their own.

Creating a more equal partnership between patients and professionals is not simply a matter of improving professionals' communication skills. Embracing a truly partnership approach to the doctor patient relationship means that both doctors and patients must change, sharing responsibility, information and decision-making. Some commentators suggest that moving to a shared decision making model of healthcare 'may be the most important change in medicine in the next decade – more important even than the arrival of the new genetics or the internet' (BMJ, 1999). The NHS Plan outlines plans for joint training for health professionals. This could include training in the skills required to ensure a shared decision-making approach to patient professional interactions (Coulter 1999). Another way of supporting patient involvement is through the use of decision aids. These provide information about which treatment options and outcomes are relevant to each person's own health status. They are available in a variety of formats, including interactive videos, computer programmes and audiotapes, as well as printed materials.

One mechanism for encouraging a more equal relationship between patients and professionals would be to involve patients in professionals' training throughout their careers. Projects are already being developed to explore how this might be put into practice. South Lewisham Primary Care Group in Lambeth, Southwark and Lewisham Health Authority has established a 'Patients As Teachers' project. Patients are involved in educating professionals about the patients' perspective on services like cardiac care and mental health. Age Concern is working with local NHS Trusts to train staff to more effectively communicate highly sensitive issues around resuscitation with older patients, relatives and their carers.

A major barrier to sharing decisions and responsibilities in healthcare is the lack of time available within the professional patient consultation. Time is an increasingly rare commodity in the NHS, particularly in primary care, and something which is keenly felt by patients and professionals alike. Increasing the amount of time patients can spend with professionals will clearly require many more doctors and nurses. Other steps may also help. Encouraging patients to take on more responsibilities for their own healthcare (see below) may not be enough on its own to free up health professionals' time. However, there is evidence that combining self-care programmes with initiatives which streamline access to services may help reduce demand at the primary care level (Rogers *et al*, 1999). A number of initiatives are already being taken in this respect, for example NHS Direct is set to become the single point of access to out-of-hours services in future. Other options for streamlining access to services should be considered, particularly the potential role that community pharmacies could play for example by enabling pharmacists to prescribe. (The evolving roles of health professionals will be explored in greater detail in IPPR's next major health policy project, *The Future Health Worker*.)

Improving patient information

Information must be improved if patients are to become genuinely empowered. Although some patients are reluctant to seek out information, particularly older patients and men, most patients generally feel very ill informed in today's NHS, both about their own diseases and treatment options and about how the NHS is performing at the national and local level.

Improving information for patients must be seen as a core health service issue, not an optional extra. The Government should therefore develop and implement a strategy to ensure high quality, timely information is available for patients.[25] A ring fenced budget should be established to help fund this strategy (although the costs and benefits of collecting and disseminating information across the entire system must also be addressed). The strategy should clarify which responsibilities should be located at the national level and which at the local. As a start, every NHS Trust, including Primary Care and Care Trust, should designate a senior member of staff responsible for ensuring that patient information is available and meets high quality standards.

Information must be improved at every stage of the patients' experience. Patient Information Leaflets (PiLs) contained in medicines packs are an important source of information but they have been criticised for being insufficiently patient friendly. Simple steps to improve PiLs include involving patients in testing draft versions, changing the order in which information is presented so that patient-focused information comes before details about the manufacturer, and ensuring pharmacists and their professional organisations work together to ensure PiLs are provided with all patient medication (Consumers Association, 2000). New ways of encouraging patients to access information that is already available must be found. Patients already have the right to see their medical records but this right is seldom exercised. Some GP practices are now offering patients the opportunity to electronically access their health records when they are in the surgery as part of a wider drive to encourage greater patient involvement in decisions and care.

Research suggests that information may be more successful in some formats than others. For example, videos have been shown to be more successful than printed information in relation to diseases like colon cancer (Meade *et al*, 1994). In general, however, the evidence about the effectiveness of patient information needs to be improved. Action is already being taken to improve the quality of cancer information (Sowden and Forbes, 2001). This approach should be applied to a broad range of different diseases and conditions. It could form a key part of current and future National Services Frameworks. In addition, the Research and Development programme should be reviewed to assess whether further primary research into the effectiveness of patient information is required. Particular attention should be paid to the needs of patients who are less likely to access and use information at present, such as older patients, men and ethnic minority groups.

Information should cover all different aspects of the condition or disease that patients want to know about. The DIPEX (Database of Individual Patient Experience) project is drawing together data on the lived experiences of patients with diseases like prostate, colorectal and breast cancer. Patients tell the story of their illness from the time the problem was first spotted, through diagnosis and treatment. Patients discuss a range of issues, including how the disease has affected their lives and their relationships with family and friends. This information is due to be made available to other patients in written, audio and visual format via the internet.

It is important to ensure that policies which seek to improve patient information do not simply reinforce a paternalistic approach . The Government aims to 'kitemark' approved websites to help patients access good quality health information over the internet. However, this policy may simply serve to reinforce assumptions that 'doctor (or government) knows best'. A more appropriate long term objective would be to ensure people have the skills and confidence to interpret information they access on the web. It has already been suggested that the school curriculum should include a 'surfing proficiency test' (Tambini, 2000). This test could include a 'check list' of questions to ask when assessing the quality of information contained in health websites, such as the source of the information and whether it has been peer reviewed. The 'checklist' could then be made available through other outlets such as GP's surgeries and NHS Direct Online.

Patients not only want information about individual diseases and conditions: they also want information about how the health service as a whole. The Government could make far better use of the information it already collects. The NHS Patient Survey, for example, interviews a cross-section of patients about how the NHS is performing. The results of this survey should be more effectively disseminated, in local surgeries, hospitals and online. This will mean accepting that the Survey will inevitably contain 'bad' as well as 'good' news: something the notoriously secretive culture of Whitehall has too often worked against in the past.

The Government recognises that its NHS Performance Indicators must be made more patient friendly. More explicit 'league tables' on both hospitals and Primary Care Groups and Trusts should be made available in future. However, this information should be collated and published by an independent body to ensure impartiality in the eyes of both patients and those working in the health service. Patients must be involved in drawing up the league tables to ensure that both the substance and style of information is as user-friendly as possible. It should be acknowledged that 'league tables' are often a very crude way of measuring and comparing public services in general and this may be particularly true of the NHS. Developing measurements which can effectively assess the quality of care being provided, or how individual hospitals and services might 'add value', will present a major challenge in future.

Lessons could be learnt from the experience of other countries in this respect. For example, the Foundation for Accountability (FACCT)[26] in the USA works with professional bodies, research agencies and patients to develop sophisticated measures of the quality of healthcare being provided. FACCT's 'measurement sets' cover a variety of issues, including the most up to date guidelines on the effective clinical management of different diseases, appropriate outcomes (such as symptom level and functioning), measures of patient education and service quality issues such as access and courtesy. A key feature of FACCT's work is to ensure the patients' perspective is included in measuring the quality of services provided. For example patients with early stage breast cancer are asked questions like: 'Did your surgeon tell you that your surgery options include either a lumpectomy or mastectomy? Did s/he explain to you the differences between the options?' If individual patients have not received important information or understood what they have been told, FACCT provides them with additional information and questions they can ask their doctor. Patients' responses are then aggregated to develop a profile of how well different surgeons score on helping their patients understand treatment options. This information is then made available to patients via the internet.

The final point is that information must be disseminated more effectively, both within the health service (for example in community pharmacies, GP's surgeries and healthy living centres) and outside it (such as in public libraries, the workplace and leisure and shopping centres). Technologies like touch screen kiosks, the internet and digital TV will provide new opportunities for disseminating health information in future. Health Improvement Programmes could be required to explain how disseminating information at the local level is to be carried forward.

Improving patient support

Some patients will be happy to access and use information on their own. However, many patients say they need support to go along with the information they receive. Research suggests that people with long term conditions, for example, want someone to talk to, particularly soon after the diagnosis made (Wilson, 1999).

There are a wide range of patient, self-help and mutual aid groups at both the local and national level. However, many patients who might value the advice and support these organisations provide are unaware that they exist. This is partly because health professionals do not know or tell patients about them. It has been suggested that patient and self-help groups need greater investment if they are to take increased roles in future. This investment should come in the form of both financial support from government and endorsement from health professionals (Wilson, 1999). Ways to improve access to patients groups should also be explored. Representatives from patients' groups could be based in one stop shops, walk in centres or community pharmacies. Money from the New Opportunities Fund could be made available for this purpose.

It may be helpful to look at what support is available to people who use other public services. In the criminal justice system, for example, victims of crime are put in touch with Victim Support. They do not have to contact or use the service if they do not wish to, but they can telephone or arrange to meet someone to talk about their experiences and the crimes they have suffered. Awareness of the service is high. Victim Support is recognised by the police to offer an important and valuable service which they themselves cannot provide and details about the service are prominently displayed in police stations.

A similar service could be developed for the NHS. The 'Patient Support Service' would provide patients with someone to talk to, for example after they have received a diagnosis. Patients could access the service by telephone or through the internet if they prefer not to contact someone face to face. The Patient Support Service would not replicate the work of existing patients groups. Instead, its purpose would be to act as a channel through which patients could be put in contact with more specialised support groups if they wish. An entirely new service would not necessarily need to be established: rather it would build on what is already happening locally. However the key would be to create a highly visible and recognisable service like Victim Support which all patients and professionals are aware of and feel confident to use. Ensuring local health services disseminate information about the new Patient Support Service would be crucial to its success. The precise functions and role of the new Patient Advocacy and Liaison Service, proposed in the NHS Plan, have yet to be fully determined. However, providing the Patient Support Service could clearly fall within PALS' remit. Another option would be to make the proposed new national body for involving patients and the public responsible for ensuring the Patient Support Service is effectively developed and implemented at the local level.

Promoting greater self-reliance

Promoting greater self-reliance amongst patients must become a key health policy objective over the coming years. Initiatives that encourage a range of self-care activities, including self-medication and the self-management of illnesses, need to be more effectively developed and implemented. The Government should build on the work of the Chief Medical Officer's Expert Patient group, which is due to report in the near future. The Expert Patient programme has been welcomed by patient groups, policy makers and industry alike. However, it should be seen as the first step in a broader process of encouraging greater self-reliance amongst all patient groups, not just those living with long term and chronic conditions.

Promoting greater self-reliance will require a significant culture shift in the attitudes of patients and professionals alike. Providing patients with more information is a crucial first step (see above) and this process should start at an early age. For example, children could be taught basic facts about the symptoms of minor ailments like the common cold, and how long these ailments are likely to last. Patients need effective support and encouragement from health professionals if they are to take on greater responsibilities for healthcare. Time is an important barrier to this happening (see above). Professionals may also lack the skills or knowledge to encourage patients to self-care. The patients' role in self-care and the self-management of illness should therefore be included as an option in both pre-qualification and in-service training (Cooper, 2001).

The cost of over the counter products has been a major barrier to promoting self-medication in the past.[27] Patients who are exempt from prescription charges – the unemployed, retired, housewives and students – are all more averse to suggestions to buy OTCs than other groups (Bradley *et al*, 1998). A number of projects have sought to address this problem. In Tyne and Wear Health Action Zone, for example, a pilot project is being established to encourage self-care amongst socially disadvantaged patients. The aim of the project is to divert the flow of conditions amenable to self-medication from the GP's surgery into the local community pharmacy. Patients who visit their local GP for minor ailments in the upper respiratory tract and gastrointestinal categories are offered the option of receiving treatment from their local pharmacy instead (although patients can still see the doctor if they choose). This treatment is free for patients who are exempt from paying prescription charges and available on direct sale to non-exempt sufferers.

One tool that has been used to promote greater self-reliance is self-care manuals. The use of these manuals has been most extensively researched in the US where their impact is usually seen in terms of whether they can help decrease demand for health services. However, evidence on the effectiveness of these manuals is both inconclusive and unlikely to be simply transferred to the UK context (Rogers *et al*, 1999). There may be more appropriate ways of encouraging self-care in the 21st century. A pilot project enabling people with mental health problems to access self-care programmes through public online centres is being piloted in some parts of the country. The aim of this programme is to provide mental health sufferers with greater privacy when exploring how they can help better care for themselves.[28]

Indeed, new technologies could help transform self-care in the future. This paper has already outlined the potential for telemedicine to increase patients' responsibilities for their own care, for example enabling patients with diabetes to take control over the management of their disease, through non-invasively monitoring their blood glucose levels, examining their feet and so on. Small, portable devices which enable patients with heart disease to monitor their condition are already available.[29] Patients with heart disease are given a 'Personal Event Recorder' to record their heart beat if they experience chest pain. The reading is then sent down a dedicated patient telephone line where trained technicians receive the reading and assess whether there are any abnormalities. If the patient needs to be admitted to hospital, the technician calls an ambulance and explains what is happening to the paramedics. The technician also call ahead to the Accident and Emergency Department of the nearest hospital to ensure they are prepared for the patient's arrival, for example by having a cardiologist available. It is vital that all patients benefit from technologies like these, not simply those patients who can afford them as is often the case at present. Patients living in disadvantaged communities are particularly likely to suffer from heart disease. The Government should therefore consider piloting the use of new technologies like cardiac monitors in more deprived areas, for example through Health Action Zones.

5. Conclusion

This report has sought to develop a more detailed understanding of what patients might want from their health services in future, outlining the available evidence of patients' attitudes towards key future trends over the next five to fifteen years. It has assessed where future patients might want to be treated, how they will want to access information and care, what they will want to be treated for and by whom. Too little attention has so far been paid to this issue, despite the fact that understanding the 'patient perspective' could have major consequences for whether and how technological advances or policy changes will be accepted and implemented in future.

The evidence outlined in this report, particularly from the qualitative research IPPR conducted during the course of the project, helps us build a picture of how different patients might access and use health services in future. Patients may include those like 'Traditional Ted', a pensioner who hates to bother anyone about his health. If Ted does get ill, he prefers to see the local practice nurse rather than trouble his GP. Ted does not like getting involved in decisions about the treatment or care he receives. So long as everything goes smoothly, he is quite happy for the doctor or nurse to take control. Ted tends not try to get any extra information about illnesses he has, although sometimes his wife tells him things she thinks he needs to know, or information she has gained from family, friends, the newspapers or TV.

'Self-sufficient Sue' is in her late sixties. Her attitude to healthcare is very different from that of Ted. Sue suffers from a long term condition and takes on considerable responsibility for her own healthcare. She participates in a self-management programme which includes some complementary therapy. If something happens that Sue cannot deal with on her own, she prefers to visit her own GP rather than the practice nurse, because he knows her medical history well. Sue is in regular contact with her local patient group, which provides her with much appreciated advice and support. She also uses the internet to contact patient groups in other countries, sometimes chatting online to fellow sufferers about the latest treatments and services that are available.

'Clued-up Carol' has two young children and she is in her early forties. She likes to know as much as she can about her health and the health of her children. She gets her information from a wide variety of sources, including family and friends, the TV, newspapers and magazines. She calls NHS Direct first if the children are unwell, particularly out of normal working hours but if she's really worried one of them is ill, she wants to see the practice nurse or GP and she does not want to wait. Carol values the advice of her local pharmacist about minor ailments and conditions. She takes a considerable role in her children's healthcare: one of them suffers from diabetes and the blood glucose monitoring kit she bought from the chemist helps her keep an eye on how things are going.

'Distant Dave', on the other hand, is not interested in health issues at all. In fact, he does everything he can to avoid contact with the NHS. If he does need to see a health professional, he likes to use the walk-in centre in town, rather than go to his local surgery where he might bump into someone he knows. Dave is twenty one and an avid internet user. He would much rather search for information on the net than ask a doctor or nurse, let alone his family or friends. Keeping fit is important to Dave. He goes to a local gym, where he recently had a series of tests on cholesterol and blood pressure as part of the annual 'Health MOT' the gym offers in partnership with his local NHS walk-in centre.

The above scenarios are, inevitably, generalisations. They represent just a few of the different types of patients who are likely to use the health service now and in the future. However they do serve to illustrate the point that a 'one size fits all' approach to the organisation and delivery of health services is no longer appropriate, if indeed it ever was. We hope this report makes a useful contribution to ensuring the NHS is a more genuinely 'patient-centred' service in the future.

Appendix: Future Patient Qualitative Research

IPPR conducted a series of focus groups to explore patient and wider public attitudes towards some of the key drivers of change during the course of the 'Future Patient' project.

Eight focus groups were conducted in total covering different age groups, gender, ethnic groups and social class. Four of the focus groups were conducted specifically with patients who had experience of either chronic or acute conditions. The focus groups were conducted in locations around England and varied in length from one and three quarter hours to three hours. Each group included between six and eight respondents who were recruited by recruitment agencies using street recruiters. They were each paid an incentive for attending the discussion group.

Focus group specifications

Group	*Age*	*Gender*	*Social Class*	*Details*	*Location*	*Length in hours*
1	18-30	M	C2DE		Timperley, Cheshire (rural)	1¾
2	18-30	F	ABC1	Afro-Caribbean	South London	1¾
3	30-50	M	C2DE	Asian	West Midlands	1¾
4	30-50	F	ABC1		West Midlands	1¾
5	30-50	F	C2DE	Inpatient in last 3 years	Birmingham	3
6	30-50	M	ABC1	Inpatient in last 3 years	Barkingside, Essex	3
7	50-65	F	C2DE	Chronic illness	Timperley Cheshire (rural)	1¾
8	50-65	M	ABC1	Chronic illness	Barkingside, Essex	1¾

Endnotes

1 These include the Nuffield Trust's report on *Policy Futures in UK Health*, the Panel in Health and Life Sciences of the *Office of Science and Technology's Foresight Programme* and numerous publications, see for example Markiner and Peckham (eds) (1998) *Clinical Futures* BMJ Books, London.

2 For further debate on the impact of the UK's ageing population, see for example the Health and Care Study Group of Age Concern's *Millennium Debate of the Age*.

3 These figures do not include any estimated years gained through future technological advances.

4 A life-course approach follows an individual's experience from conception to death in order to avoid a false dichotomy between adult lifestyle and early life or between biological and social risk.

5 This issue has been discussed in greater detail in New, B (2000) *What Business is the NHS in? Establishing the boundary of a health care system's responsibility* IPPR, London.

6 A number of recent reports have discussed this issue in detail. See for example Lenaghan J (1998) *Brave New NHS? The impact of the new genetics on the health service* IPPR, London and Zimmern R and Cook C (2000) *Genetics and Health: Policy issues for genetic science and their implications for health and health services* The Nuffield Trust Genetics Scenarios Project, Nuffield Trust, London.

7 See for example the House of Commons Select Committee (1995) *Human Genetics: the Science and its Consequences* and the work of the Human Genetics Committee.

8 *Health Service Journal* 15 March 2001.

9 The stereotype of the British patiently waiting in queues is perhaps nowhere more aptly illustrated than in the long waits for healthcare experienced in this country. Indeed, waiting may be a peculiarly British disease: waiting for health care is simply not an issue in many other European countries. Comparisons between key trends experienced in the UK and other European countries will be explored through the international wing of the 'Future Patient' project which is being co-ordinated by the Picker Institute, Europe.

10 www.doh.gov.uk/nhsperformanceindicators

11 www.drfoster.co.uk

12 This programme is being lead by the Chief Medical Officer and is due

to report in the near future.

13 It is thought that as many as half of all patients with chronic conditions end up using their medicines in a way that is not fully effective. Estimates of the number of hospital admissions that are due to problems with medicines typically range from six to ten per cent.

14 It has been suggested that there are three models doctors use to consult with their patients (although the differences between these different models are clearly more subtle in reality). Firstly, the paternalistic model of healthcare, where the doctor decides what to do. Secondly, the informed patient model, where the patient decides what to do after the doctor has explained the available options. Thirdly, the shared decision making model, where the doctor and patient decide what to do together.

15 There are 5,000 people on the People's Panel. They are ordinary members of the public aged 16 years and over who are representative of the UK population as a whole in terms of age, gender, region and a range of other demographic indicators (Cabinet Office, 2000).

16 It is important to note that most studies of telemedicine have so far explored issues of cost-effectiveness and the attitude of the health professionals involved in using the technology, rather than focusing on patients' views. Several problems have been identified with the evidence on patient attitudes that does exist. Telemedicine trials tend to use small samples of volunteers, which could lead to bias, and to take place in locations which may have little relevance to the wider system of health care, such as prisons. Few of the studies go into any depth about what 'patient satisfaction' really means or attempt to understand the reasons why patients were satisfied or dissatisfied with teleconsultations. The studies also fail to explore what happens to patient satisfaction over time, thereby opening up the possibility that the 'novelty' value of the technology results in a positive bias (Mair and Whitten, 2000).

17 The NHS Plan has already proposed making NHS Direct the single point of access for out of hours services. This raises the possibility that NHS Direct could eventually become the first port of call for all primary care services in future.

18 MORI conducted a representative survey of 1000 members of the Government's People's Panel on public attitudes towards the use of genetic information, the results of which were published in March 2001. A booster sample of interviews with Black and Asian respondents was held to ensure a sufficiently large base size for

separate analysis.

19 Speech by the Secretary of State for Health, Institute of Human Genetics, International Centre for Life, Newcastle Upon Tyne, 19 April 2001.

20 HON is a not for profit organisation which carries out polls of medical and health related internet users. 3,276 Web users took part in HON's poll in October-November 1999. 58 per cent of respondents were from North America and 28 per cent were from Europe. The remaining 14 per cent were from South America, Oceania, Asia, Africa, the Middle East and Central America. www.hon.ch/survey

21 It is important to note that use of the internet is a fast moving area and any figures which indicate levels of access tend to become quickly out date.

22 *Time for Common Sense* Conservative Party Manifesto, May 2001

23 *Ambitions for Britain* Labour Party Manifesto, May 2001

24 *Freedom, Justice, Honesty* Liberal Democrat Party Manifesto, May 2001

25 Some of these recommendations have been made elsewhere. See for example Coulter *et al* (1999).

26 FACCT (www.facct.org) is a not for profit organisation based in Portland, Oregon. See Odyssey (*The Glaxo Wellcome Journal of Innovation in Helathcare*) Vol 6, Issue 2, 2000.

27 The outcome of the recent court case on the Resale Price Maintenance (which means it is no longer legal to set minimum resale prices on branded OTC medicines) could lead to a substantial reduction in the cost of OTCs in future.

28 *Health Service Journal* 4 January 2001

29 www.lifewatchinc.com

Bibliography

Beck U (1992) *Risk Society*, Sage Publications, London

Bell J (1998), 'The human genome' in Marinker M and Peckham M (eds), *Clinical Futures*, BMJ Books

Boudioni M and McPherson K (2000) 'Cancer patients information needs and information seeking behaviour: in depth interview study' *British Medical Journal* 320: 909-913.

Bowling A, Stramer K, Dickinson E, Windson J, Bond M (1997) 'Evaluation of specialists' outreach clinics in general practice in England: process and acceptability to patients, specialists and general practitioners' *Journal of Epidemiology and Community Health* 51: 52-61.

Blenkinsopp A and Bradley C (1996) 'Patients, society and the increase of self-medication' *British Medical Journal* 312: 629-640.

Bradley C, Riaz A, Tobias R, Kenkre J and Dassu D (1998) 'Patient attitudes to OTC drugs and possible professional responses to self-medication' *Family Practice* 15 (1): 44-50.

British Council (1998) Obesity: A Global Challenge, International Seminar 17 October 1998, Rowett Research Institute, Aberdeen

British Medical Journal (1999), Editorial, 18 Sept 1999

Cabinet Office (2000) *Open all hours?* Results from the People's Panel, Issue 5.

Calman K (1998) *On the State of Public Health 1997* The Stationery Office, London

Central IT Unit (1998) *Electronic Government: the View from the Queue* Cabinet Office.

Chapple A, Rogers A, Macdonald W and Sergison M (2000) 'Patients perceptions of changing professional boundaries and the future of nurse led services' *Primary Health Care Research and Development* 1: 51-59.

Cooper L, Coote A, Davies A and Jackson C (1995) *Voices Off: Tackling the democratic deficit in health* IPPR, London

Cooper J (2001) *Partnerships for Successful Self-Management, The Living with Long-term Illness (Lill) Project Report* Long-term Medical Conditions Alliance, London

Coote A and Kendall L (2000) 'Well women and medicine men: gendering the health policy agenda' in Coote A (ed) *New Gender Agenda*, IPPR

Consumers' Association (2000) *Patient information leaflets: sick notes?* London

Coulter A (1999) 'Paternalism or Partnership? Patients have grown up – and there's no going back' *British Medical Journal* 319: 719-720.

Coulter A, Entwistle V and Gilbert, D (1999) 'Sharing decisions with patients: is the information good enough' *British Medical Journal* 318

Dahlgren G and Whitehead M (1991) *Policies and Strategies to Promote Social Equity in Health* Institute for Futures Studies, Mimeo, Stockholm

Dargie C (1999) *Demographics and Ageing, Policy Futures for UK Health* The Nuffield Trust

Dennis T and Owens D (2000) 'Transforming local care' *Journal of Telemedicine and Telecare* 6, Supplement 1, 2000

Department of Health (1998) *The National Survey of NHS Patients: General Practice.*

Department of Health (2000a) *The NHS Plan: A plan for investment, A plan for reform* The Stationery Office, London.

Department of Health (2000b) *Shaping the future NHS: Long Term Planning for Hospitals and Related Services* Consultation Document on the Findings of the National Beds Inquiry, The Stationery Office, London

Department of Health (2000c) *Pharmacy in the Future – Implementing the NHS Plan, A programme for pharmacy in the National Health Service* The Stationery Office, London

Department for Trade and Industry (1999) *IT is for All* The Stationery Office, London.

Edwards A, Elwyn G and Gwyn R (1999), 'General practice registrar responses to use of different risk communication tools in simulated consultation: a focus group study' *British Medical Journal* 7212, 18 Sept 1999

Edwards L (2001) *The Future of Healthcare: the Patient Perspective in England* IPPR, London (unpublished)

East Anglian Cancer Unit (1997) *Report of Cancer Incidence and Prevalence Projections* Macmillan Cancer Relief, London

Economic Trends (2001) Office for National Statistics, April 2001

Gilchrist C (1999) *Turning your back on us: older people and the NHS* Age Concern England, London

Hassell K, Noyce P R, Rogers A, Harris J, and Wilkinson J (1997) 'A Pathway to the GP: the pharmaceutical "consultation" as the first port of call in primary health care' *Family Practice* 14 (6): 498-502

Hills J (2001) *Taxation for the Enabling State* CASE Paper 41, Centre for the Analysis of Social Exclusion, LSE, London

House of Lords (2000) *Select Committee on Science and Technology Report on Complementary and Alternative Medicine*

ICM poll (1999) reported in 'Poll points to lift- off for Internet *The Guardian* 11 January 1999

Illman J (2000) *The expert patient* ABPI, London

Independent Inquiry into Inequalities in Health (1998) Chairman: Sir Donald Acheson, The Stationery Office, London

IPPR (1998) *Rights and Responsibilities* Draft report of public consultation for Policy Forum on the Future of Health and Healthcare, IPPR, London

Lee K (1999) *Global Context, A review of priority global health issues for the UK* Policy Futures for UK Health, The Nuffield Trust, London.

Lenaghan J (1998) *Brave New NHS? The impact of the new genetics on the health service* IPPR, London.

Lenaghan J (1999) *The National Health Service, Today and Tomorrow* Report of Community Issue Groups, IPPR.

Mair F and Whitten P (2000) 'Systematic review of studies of patient satisfaction with telemedicine' *British Medical Journal* 320: 1517-1520

Marinker M (1998) 'Looking and leaping' in Marinker M and Peckham M (eds) *Clinical Futures* BMJ Books

May C, Gash L, Ellis N, Atkinson, T, Mair F, Smith C, Pidd S, and Esmail A (2000) 'Telepsychiatry evaluation in the North West of England: preliminary results of a qualitative study' *Journal of Telemedicine and Telecare* 6, Supplement 1.

Meade C, McKinney W and Barnas G (1994), 'Educating patients with limited literacy skills: the effectiveness of printed and videotaped material about colon cancer' *American Journal of Public Health* 84, (1).

Mihill C (2000) *Shaping tomorrow: issues facing general practice in the new millennium* BMA, London

Mitchell J (2000) 'Increasing the cost effectiveness of telemedicine by embracing e-health' *Journal of Telemedicine and Telecare* 6, Supplement 1

New B (2000) *What Business is the NHS is? Establishing the boundary of health care system's responsibility* IPPR, London

NOP (1999) Internet User Profile Study: Wave 7, presented to DTI February 1999

Pahl R (1999) 'Social Trends: the social context of healthy living' *Policy Futures for UK Health* The Nuffield Trust, London

Palmer S (1999) *The Physical Environment, Policy Futures for UK Health* The Nuffield Trust, London

Paterson C and Britten N (1999) ''Doctors can't help much': the search for an alternative' *British Journal of General Practice* 49; (445), 626-629.

Putnam R (2001) *Bowling Alone* Simon Schuster, London

Rashid A, Jagger C and Goodyer L (1996) 'Views of Asians and non Asians on sources of drug information and the desirability for medication to be made available over the counter' *British Journal of General Practice* 46 (411): 609-610.

Rawlinson, Kelly and Whittlestone (2000) *Telemedicine – The Virtual Hospital or Virtually no Change?*

Robert G (1999) 'Science and Technology, Trends and Issues forward to 2015: Implications for Healthcare' *Policy Future for UK Health* Technical Series, Nuffield Trust, London.

Rogers A, Hassell K, and Nicolaas G (1999) *Demanding patients? Analysing the Use of Primary Care* OU Press, Buckingham

Social Exclusion Unit (1999) *Report of Policy Action Team 15: Information Technology* National Strategy for Neighbourhood Renewal.

Sowden, A and Forbes, C (2001) 'Patient information' *Health Service Journal* 1 March 2001

Stroetmann K, Gretzmacher P and Stroetmann V (2000) 'Improving quality of life for dialysis patients through telecare' *Journal of Telemedicine and Telecare* 6, Supplement 1.

Tambini D, 'A Surfing Proficiency Test' *Times Educational Supplement* Friday 15 December 2000.

Taylor D and Esmail A (1999) 'Retrospective analysis of census data on general practitioners who qualified in South Asia: who will replace them as they retire?' *British Medical Journal* 318: 306-310.

Vincent and Furnham (1996) 'Why do patients turn to complementary medicine? An empirical study' *British Journal of Clinical Psychology* 35: 37-38.

Walker J, Brooksby A, McInerny J, and Taylor A (1998) 'Patient perception of hospital care: building confidence, faith and trust' *Journal of Nursing Management* 6: 193-200.

WHO (1998) *Obesity: Preventing and Managing the Global Epidemic* Report of a World Health Organisation consultation on obesity, Geneva

Wilkinson R G (1996) *Unhealthy Societies: the Affliction of Inequality* Routledge, London.

Williams S, Weinman J, and Dale J (1998) 'Doctor patient communication and patient satisfaction: a review' *Family Practice* 15: 480-492.

Williams S, Calnan M (1991) 'Key determinants of consumer satisfaction with general practice' *Family Practice* 8: 237-242.

Wilson J (1999), 'Acknowledging the expertise of patients and their organisations' *British Medical Journal* 7212, 18 September 1999.

Wyatt J C (1998) 'Four Barriers to Realising the Information Revolution in Health Care', in Lenaghan J (ed) (1998) *Rethinking IT and Health* IPPR, London.

Zimmern R and Cook C, 2000 *Genetics and Health: Policy issues for genetic science and their implications for health and health services* The Nuffield Trust Genetics Scenarios Project, Nuffield Trust, London.